The Cultural Context
of Health, Illness,
and Medicine

The Cultural Context of Health, Illness, and Medicine

Second Edition

Elisa J. Sobo and Martha O. Loustaunau

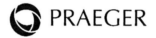 PRAEGER

AN IMPRINT OF ABC-CLIO, LLC
Santa Barbara, California • Denver, Colorado • Oxford, England

Library of Congress Cataloging-in-Publication Data

Sobo, Elisa Janine, 1963–
    The cultural context of health, illness, and medicine / Elisa J. Sobo and Martha O. Loustaunau. — 2nd ed.
        p. ; cm.
    Martha Loustaunau is first named author on previous edition.
    Includes bibliographical references and index.
    ISBN 978–0–313–37760–0 (hard copy : alk. paper) — ISBN 978–0–313–37785–3 (pbk. : alk. paper) — ISBN 978–0–313–37761–7 (eISBN)
1. Medical anthropology. 2. Social medicine. I. Loustaunau, Martha O., 1938– II. Title.
    [DNLM: 1. Cultural Competency—United States. 2. Anthropology—United States.
3. Attitude to Health—ethnology—United States. 4. Cultural Diversity—United States.
5. Delivery of Health Care—United States. W 21 S677c 2010]
GN296.L68   2010
306.4′61—dc22   2010014928

ISBN: 978–0–313–37760–0
ISBN (paperback): 978–0–313–37785–3
EISBN: 978–0–313–37761–7

14 13 12 11 10   1 2 3 4 5

This book is also available on the World Wide Web as an eBook.
Visit www.abc-clio.com for details.

Praeger
An Imprint of ABC-CLIO, LLC

ABC-CLIO, LLC
130 Cremona Drive, P.O. Box 1911
Santa Barbara, California 93116-1911

This book is printed on acid-free paper ∞

Manufactured in the United States of America

Portions of the text were reproduced from *Caring for Patients from Different Cultures*, 4th edition, by Geri-Ann Galanti. Philadelphia: University of Pennsylvania Press, 2008. Used by permission.

Contents

Preface to Second Edition

People of all cultures confront illness, disability, and death: everyone gets sick, many become disabled, and ultimately everyone dies. Systems of health care thus exist within every culture, as a **cultural universal**. The ways in which we perceive and interpret health and illness, and seek and deliver care, however, are inextricably bound up with cultural norms, beliefs, and values, as well as by social structure and environmental conditions. This book focuses on the various dimensions of this relationship, as did its first edition.

However, times have changed. When the first edition was written, the cultural competence movement had not yet emerged. Today, it is well-established. Yet the need for change persists. The new edition continues to press for positive modifications, but it also now urges a more sophisticated approach: Culture is a far more multifaceted human process than "recipe" or checklist models allow.

Moreover, political, economic, and sociocultural contexts have shifted, as have the ways that we handle health, illness, medicine, and health care delivery. For example, cultural ideas regarding complementary and alternative medicine, genetic testing, use of technology for medical communication, and even the value of being a multicultural society have evolved. Health challenges themselves have evolved, both for better (for instance with new drug discoveries, such as for treatment of HIV/AIDS) and for worse (with emerging infectious diseases, increasing health disparities, etc.). The second edition of this text reflects such changes, and includes updates on concepts, theories, and research and development. As a result, the systems perspective has been strengthened. As well, greater appreciation of cultural evolution's role in health care's evolution is promoted. Several new sections also have been added, incorporating relevant new information, including on globalization, stress, health care consumerism, reform, and technology. The discussion questions at each chapter's end have, accordingly, been updated.

Throughout the revision process, our goal has mainly been to keep the text relevant, and so where newer scholarship simply corroborated older observations, especially those now considered seminal, the text remains as it was. Older references retained therefore do not index a dated text; rather, they reveal to readers the historical depth of certain patterns or ideas.

Continuity also is maintained in the way that the book continues to promote the transdisciplinary perspective that brought us together in the early 1990s when we realized the need for a text examining the multicultural context of health, illness, and medicine from a combined sociological and anthropological standpoint. Separate disciplines are often too narrow in their focus and interpretations; the use of transdisciplinary viewpoints offers a broader, more illuminating perspective. The subdisciplines of medical sociology and medical anthropology address health, illness, and medicine from very similar, sometimes overlapping, and yet often distinctive perspectives. Although there has been much cross-disciplinary fertilization and borrowing, each discipline has its specific focus and terminology. This text draws on the strengths of each discipline.

Although, in the interest of space, with the second as with the first edition we have had to streamline the bibliography and be selective regarding topics covered and level of detail, we still include ideas and research from numerous perspectives within our respective disciplines, and discussions on current (often controversial) issues. Our purpose is still to generate in readers the motivation and capability to recognize and understand socially and culturally relevant factors that influence our views and constructions of health, illness, and healing, as well as of science and medicine.

Given this goal, from the start our project was not one that we could carry out on our own. While we, alone, are responsible for this work, shortcomings and all, we are indebted to colleagues for their insightful and critical comments and suggestions, and for kindly permitting us to quote from their works. Although we do not have the space to name all who contributed, those to whom we owe thanks, beginning with the first edition, include Helen Ball, Robert Echenberg, S. Malia Fullerton, Geri-Ann Galanti, H. Jack Geiger, Kate Hill, Pat Hippo, Jill Kerr, Tamara Kohn, Terry Meyer, Mark Nathan, Milagros Pena, Billy Reeves, Andrew Russell, Charles Sanders, Robert Simpson, Loudell Snow, Adina Sobo, and Wenda Trevathan, not to mention our long-suffering spouses, Joaquin Loustaunau and Harvey Smallman, who sweated through the project with us. For the second edition, we give special thanks to educators, students, and health professionals who embraced the first edition and advocated the present update.

Introduction

This book brings together medical sociology and medical anthropology in an effort to provide a useful resource for developing and delivering relevant and effective health care. Long traditions of research on medically related topics exist in both anthropology and sociology. But the formal subdisciplines of medical sociology and medical anthropology began to emerge as such only in the mid-1900s. This introduction reviews their emergence and then outlines a chapter-by-chapter road map for the journey we intend to take using insights from each of these subfields.

A BRIEF DISCIPLINARY HISTORY

MEDICAL ANTHROPOLOGY

Medical anthropology did not stand out from general anthropology until well after World War II, when it received impetus and support from applied work in the arena of international public health, much of which was government funded. Many saw the field in the 1960s as a "practice discipline" (Good 1994), dedicated to the service of improving public health in economically poor nations.

Despite the fact that this recent involvement with public health was key to its formal emergence, medical anthropology has old roots. These extend in two general directions, reflecting two kinds of anthropology: biological or what used to be called "physical," and sociocultural. And while some anthropologists from both camps followed the public health line when it came along, others kept their interests academic.

Indeed, there was great debate within the discipline regarding the merits of either angle, with many asserting that applied work was inferior or somehow tainted anthropology's academic dignity. Even George Foster, a key founding figure in U.S. medical anthropology, had to work through ambivalences here. "We were trained to despise applied anthropology," he once said, recalling that he did not join the Society for Applied Anthropology until 1950; until then "I would have nothing of it" (Foster 2000, quoted in Kemper 2006). Today, however, that divide has been recognized as wrong-headed. Theory can really be tested only when applied, and good applied work hinges on a strong theoretical grounding.

Most medical anthropologists take somewhat of a systems approach in their work in any case. Among biological medical anthropologists, major areas of study include diet, nutrition, and evolutionary adaptation. In the sociocultural branch of anthropology, which is the branch this book draws most upon, there has been a longstanding ethnographic interest in medical practices, knowledge, and beliefs, generally viewed as part of the total culture of peoples studied (Foster 1978; for more on early history, see also Sobo in press).

In the later part of the twentieth century, however, many socioculturally oriented anthropologists turned toward symbolic analysis of illness representations and explanations, in both medical knowledge and popular social representations of the body and of diseases, such as AIDS. A trend toward strengthening worn ties between the biological and sociocultural branches of anthropology also took root. Of late, interest in human-environment interaction has increased, in tandem with a boost in popular interest in a "greener" lifestyle.

Also today, persons' socioculturally situated "subjectivities" or inner lives and experiences are attracting attention, as are issues related to global flows, for instance of technologies, medicines—and even patients. The critical perspective, which takes global and local political and economic arrangements into account, has come to be an expected aspect of medical anthropological work. Indeed, social variables have been increasingly factored in as the links between sociology and anthropology have been strengthened (e.g., Auge and Herzlich 1995). Medical anthropology, however, has only recently entered into medical school curricula on a wide scale, and more often than not this is in the problematic arena of "cultural competence" (more of which later; see Chapter 7).

MEDICAL SOCIOLOGY

Medical sociology's history is quite different. Reflecting positivist values, the subdiscipline was situated within the framework of the scientific medical model from the start; it saw medicine as part of a functioning social system, and illness as a form of deviance (e.g., Parsons 1951). Changes in morbidity and mortality after World War II, the rise of preventive medicine, the establishment of modern psychiatry, and administrative needs contributed to medical sociology's rise (Coe 1978). Medical sociologists gained acceptance and credibility through applied work from within the medical field, finding faculty positions in medical schools. There was, however, little or no recognition that "medicine" includes diverse systems, all of which are influenced by the cultural contexts in which they are actualized (Gerhardt 1989).

In addition to applied sociology within the medical field, sociological interests essentially cover four broad categories: the relationship between environment and health and illness; health and illness behaviors; the relationship of health care practitioners with their patients; and the health care system or the organization of health care delivery (Weiss and Lonnquist, 1994, 6). Further, the concept of culture has become more significant in medical sociology. Like anthropologists, many sociologists now consider biomedicine both a product of culture and a culture in itself.

While sociologists still focus on the dominant medical systems in both Europe and America, since the early 1980s medical sociology has expanded and broadened in scope, becoming an academic discipline with a focus on practical application. As noted by Cockerham, "Not only have the numbers of medical sociologists continually increased, but also the scope of matters pertinent to medical sociology has clearly broadened as issues of health, illness, and medicine have become a medium through which general issues and concerns about society have been expressed" (2010, 7). Both the sociological and medical fields have recognized that they have mutual interests that converge. Medical sociologists of the twenty-first century are most concerned with how the discipline increases our knowledge and understanding of the "complex relationship between social factors and health" (7).

A CHOICE OF TERMS

Much research in medical sociology and anthropology originates from within the perspective of European and American scientifically and, particularly, biologically (and, increasingly, genetically) based medicine. This system is generally referred to as the "true" or benchmark medical system. In comparison, other medical systems, from Chinese acupuncture to Caribbean bush medicine, are often dismissed and devalued without consideration or understanding of possible functions or benefits. The dominant medical system often is referred to by such terms as "modern medicine," "cosmopolitan medicine," "Western medicine," "clinical medicine," "mainstream medicine," and "biomedicine." Each term has its pros and cons.

In this text, we have chosen to use the term "biomedicine" when discussing the dominant medical system, since "bio" suggests that health and wellness are physiological issues, which are the focus of the biomedical model. We do note that other medicines may also be biologically grounded (albeit perhaps in biologies that differ from the dominant U.S. or European version). We will refer to our subdisciplines as "medical," because professional associations in the United States use the label, and with the understanding that the subjects covered go far beyond the generic term of identification.

"Science" is a term that can also be problematic. Many systems claim "scientific" systematized knowledge derived from observation and study. However, our use of "science" in relation to medicine refers to the series of systematic, organized steps that ensures maximum objectivity as well as consistency in research. This system, known as the scientific method, has produced discoveries and inventions from antibiotics and surgical success to genetic engineering and space travel. It is not, of course, value free: Recent investigations have called into question the objectivity of the research process, the nature of evidentiary claims, and so on (see, for instance, Lambert 2006; Lipman 2000; Sobo 2009; see also Lambert, Gordon, and Bogdan-Lovis 2006).

Another terminological problem with which we have had to come to grips involves the national focus of the text. While it is true that much of what we say has implications for other economically developed nations, including most Western European nations, most of the research we cite in relation to biomedicine is written from a U.S. perspective. So, the generalizations that can be made from this work notwithstanding, when we refer to "our" society, we are referring to the United States. We use the term "America" to refer to the United States advisedly: America really is the name of a continent group, and there are many nations in the Americas.

One last problem with terminology involves the distinctions among the definitions of "illness," "sickness," and "disease." While "disease" refers to the medical or pathological source of a problem, "illness" generally refers to the individual experience of being ill.

Sociologists use the word "sickness" for describing a social response to unwellness as a form of deviance. Unwellness requires a person to take on, at least temporarily, a social role, referring to societal expectations about the attitudes and behavior of the "sick" person. In anthropological jargon, the term "sickness" can be used to draw attention to the social-structural causes of unwellness.

Notwithstanding such technical distinctions (and regarding their history, see Parsons 1951; Cockerham 2010, 158), illness and sickness are often used interchangeably. We have attempted to use them appropriately, but recognize that meanings may become blurred and have therefore often used the term "illness" as a general designation.

THE SOCIOCULTURAL APPROACH: A CHOICE BLEND

One of medical anthropology's founders, George Foster, in his discussion of the disciplines of sociology and anthropology, noted the value of combining them in order to learn more by providing a broader perspective: "Precisely because we ask different questions, seek out different data, and come to conclusions that reflect our professional biases, our total understanding of medical and health phenomena is richer and more varied than if the task were left to a single discipline. We are in complementary, and not competitive, lines of work. We learn from each other, and we teach each other. Our society needs both of us" (1978, 10–11). As a sociologist (Loustaunau) and an anthropologist (Sobo), we agree.

The basic focus of this text is therefore to examine the role of cultural differences in defining and dealing with health and illness, and to investigate the health-related factors that link humanity cross-culturally through common needs, using our two related disciplines. Each perspective gives us specific knowledge and understanding of the many elements that make up health, illness, and medical behaviors and systems. Both perspectives recognize how an appreciation for and an understanding of cultural diversity as well as commonalities are essential for developing a unified and effective system of health care delivery in our distinctly multicultural nation. And, in doing so, neither perspective will let slip from view the social-structural factors that contribute to health inequities, whether locally or globally.

Health care in the United States is based upon the biomedical model (defined earlier). Until recently, the biomedical model has not supported cultural awareness and sensitivity in health care delivery, whether for acute problems, for chronic conditions, or in recovery or rehabilitation. It has also, until recently, given little recognition to alternative healing systems and beliefs that exist side by side with biomedicine and that are often used instead of or in conjunction with mainstream care.

At the same time, America has grown increasingly culturally diverse. Drawing from both sociology and anthropology, we examine how cultural backgrounds, diverse beliefs and values, and societal structures are related to physical and mental health. What are the various ways people perceive health and illness, and how do those perceptions affect related behaviors? What political and economic issues are involved? How and why does the health system that is meant to care for all of us incorporate or exclude those cultural aspects of our identities that play such a large part in our health status? How can we improve this system's ability to provide the best possible quality of life for those it serves? And why does culture matter?

THE TEXT: A PREVIEW

In Chapter 1, we examine the concept of culture, and establish its significance with relation to health and illness. The role of culture is explored in terms of identity and behavior, and its consequent links to health, disease, and illness.

Issues of ethnocentrism, cultural relativism, and multiculturalism are addressed in relation to social and political controversy, and the difficulties of finding a balance between diversity and unity are explored. We suggest that medical care that excludes diverse cultural factors and considerations falls short of addressing human needs that must be met.

Chapter 2 explores the influence of social structure and related variables in causes of and approaches to health and illness in our multicultural society. The pivotal roles of kinship and family, ethnicity, gender, and social class are shown to shape how both consumers and providers perceive and deal with illness and maintain health. These variables are also examined as sources for and causes of illness, and of discrimination in and barriers to care seeking and treatment—some of which support persisting health inequities.

The different stages of our lives entail different health and illness challenges and require different approaches to care and coping. Chapter 3 addresses birth and childhood, adolescence, adulthood, and old age; it investigates the many and diverse cultural issues associated with these life stages. Issues of sexuality, maternal-child health, and death are also discussed in relation to cultural context, focusing on their implications for health care on the personal and structural levels.

All cultures have socially sanctioned as well as limited, marginalized, quasi, and auxiliary modalities of treatment. Chapter 4 defines and discusses a number of these modalities. It includes an examination of intercultural differences and commonalities, and of ways in which many of these modalities may be complementary. Dangerous therapies and quackery are also discussed as they relate to cultural relativity, individual choice, and legal concerns. We stress the need for education of both providers and consumers.

Chapters 5 and 6 examine how the U.S. health care system evolved from its diverse folk roots into the now dominant biomedical culture. Various cultural contributions and institutional values, as well as technological developments and the emergence of powerful political and economic interests, have all played roles in the formation of the American health care system and the resulting dominance of biomedicine in it.

Biomedicine is characterized both as a part of the larger culture, reflecting its mainstream norms, values, and beliefs, and as a culture in itself, based on the scientific model, with its own language, structure, and, again, norms, values, and beliefs. Biomedical culture also is viewed in terms of various elements, including service versus profit orientations in care delivery, changing patient- or client-practitioner relationships, ethical concerns as they are fueled by increasing costs and new technological and service innovations, pressures for (and against) reform, and globalization processes. All reveal the limitations of the biomedical paradigm.

Chapter 7 centers on problems of cross-cultural communication. Besides language differences, ethnocentrism too must be overcome.

This chapter discusses cultural sensitivity, using examples, and describes various techniques by which health care workers can more effectively serve culturally diverse populations.

We tie the lessons of previous chapters together in Chapter 8, which discusses, by way of example, the connections between culture and HIV/AIDS. We focus particularly on HIV because cultural attitudes, perceptions, beliefs, and norms are so very important in the transmission, prevention, and treatment of such health threats. However, the lessons can be generalized or extended to most other health challenges. Recent treatment of so-called swine flu exemplifies this.

Chapter 8 also suggests how the various modalities and themes addressed throughout the text might be combined and integrated to provide more sensitive, effective, humane, and accessible health care overall. The need for cooperation and inclusion rather than narrowly focused and competitive models is stressed. Issues of cost, power, relativism and diversity, communication, and respect for human rights must be considered with the aim of moving toward a more realistic model of health care delivery in increasingly pluralistic contexts.

GOALS AND CONSIDERATIONS

This book was not written to answer all of the very difficult questions raised by the challenging problems of health care delivery in a multicultural society. It does, however, emphasize the links that have been identified between culture, social structure, and the health and well-being of a population. What those links are, and their role in the evolution and provision of just and humane health care, is a main focus of this volume. Increasing cultural diversity, burgeoning technology, health care disparities, and global health issues are forcing change in the system in spite of economic and political resistance.

Beyond sharing with readers background information on this context and the ways it affects and is implicated in biomedicine, we ask how to retain and utilize knowledge of cultural diversity in biomedical care delivery while maintaining a sense of unity in the face of common difficulties of suffering across cultures. Inclusion of an understanding and appreciation of cultural diversity and commonality in the education of health care providers, as well as of patients, is vital and essential for creating an effective health care system.

CHAPTER 1

The Concept of Culture

GOAL: Explain and analyze the concept of culture and identify its components and elements through anthropological and sociological approaches.

GOAL: Examine ethnocentrism, cultural relativism, and multiculturalism and become aware of their meanings, controversies, impacts, and significance for health care in the twenty-first century.

If anything was made to be taken for granted, it is culture.

(Gallagher and Subedi 1995, 4)

Culture is present in all aspects of life. And yet, until faced with a contrasting culture that challenges the basis of our beliefs, values, and identity, we generally take our own culture for granted. In the area of health care provision, cultural diversity and the experience of contrasts is increasing. This affects the relationships of patients and providers and the outcomes of their interactions, as well as the relationships between and among providers themselves. Effective and humane health care demands that we all learn more about culture—what it is, how it functions, and its relevance for our interactions and their outcomes.

WHAT IS CULTURE?

In attempting to understand and analyze health and illness in any society, individual behaviors, interactions, and social structures must be placed within a cultural context. A **culture** is, put briefly, a society's shared, learned knowledge base and behavior patterns. A **society** consists of people who interact together, guided by their culture.

Societies have organizational or **social structures**, by which various roles, statuses, and systems such as marriage, education, and work are arranged in patterns of relationships to each other and passed down through generations. Social structures are more, or less, hierarchical depending on the cultures that support them. Importantly, social structures do not stand alone: Today more than ever, societies are linked together in a complex global system (see Chapter 2).

Culture guides how people live, what they generally believe and value, how they communicate, and what are their habits, customs, and tastes. It guides the ways people meet the various needs of society: how goods and services are produced and distributed; how power and decision making are designated, what god or gods are represented (if any). Culture prescribes rituals, art forms, entertainment, and customs of daily living. Most certainly, the ways in which we interpret and perceive health and illness and our choices in providing and seeking care are influenced by our culture.

Culture is in some ways then a kind of knowledge base that we use and act on. Some of this knowledge is **declarative** in that it consists of apparently factual information ("Mint tea is good for digestion"). Some of it is **procedural**, or how-to information ("Boil a handful of mint leaves in water until the water turns dark; pour this water into a cup through a strainer and drink when cool enough"). Cultural knowledge of both kinds exists in relation to all realms of existence, including subsistence or food production, economics, kinship, government or the maintenance of order, religion, gender, leisure, and health and illness. Importantly, cultural knowledge can be changed or adapted by its users to fit new conditions. A group's culture is always evolving as the life circumstances of the group change (see Wedenoja and Sobo 1997).

Cultures are composed of norms, values, and beliefs. These are the rules of the game—the guidelines for action. **Norms** set standards for appropriate behavior. These standards are based on cultural **values**, or principles by which members of a culture determine what is right and wrong, good and bad. **Beliefs** are what a culture deems to be true or false.

Norms, values, and beliefs are made real through action, in word and deed. Members of a culture generally strive to enforce cultural norms, either informally, or formally through law. When norms are violated, cultural punishments may be invoked, by the individual who judges his or her own behavior self-reflexively, by his or her community, or by both. Depending on the nature of the violation, punishment may entail anything from light scorn to execution (whether self-imposed, as suicide, or imposed by others). In addition to varying across cultures, norms, values, and beliefs also vary over time. Importantly, cultural evolution is due not only to outside forces but to the ongoing negotiations by its members.

DOMINANT CULTURES AND SUBCULTURES

The United States is considered a **pluralistic** society in which multiple cultures ideally exist side by side in harmony. Basic institutions are also shared by all, including the political, economic, and legal systems as well as a common language. Pluralism as an ideal, however, is greatly endangered by prejudice, discrimination, and selective immigration policies. Pluralism is also qualified. Where multiple cultures mix or meet, as they do in the United States, the society must promote some sense of consensus among all members concerning basic norms, beliefs, and values. The mainstream or **dominant culture** (sometimes referred to as a **core** culture) is the one whose norms, values, language, structures, and institutions tend to predominate.

In the United States, the dominant culture has typically been white due to colonization by peoples of Western European origins. Williams (1970) identified 15 of what he considered to be major themes and value orientations representative of the dominant culture in the United States—orientations still relevant today, for the most part.

1. Personal achievement and success
2. Hard work and productivity
3. Humanitarianism and support of the "underdog"
4. Orientation toward moral judgments of events and situations
5. Pragmatism, or practicality and efficiency

6. Progress toward a better life
7. Materialism and consumerism
8. Equality for all
9. Freedom and individual autonomy
10. Outward conformity, as in dress, recreation, housing, and political expression
11. Science as a tool of mastery over the environment
12. Nationalism and loyalty to that which is "American"
13. Democratic principles and belief in everyone having a voice in political matters
14. Individual importance and responsibility
15. Racism and the idea of group superiority

Some of those themes indicate conflicting values, such as the value of equality (the idea that all people have a right to health care) and an emphasis on racism and related group superiority (which results in denial of care to those without insurance or who cannot pay—generally members of various disadvantaged racial and ethnic groups and most recently undocumented immigrants).

Contradictions like these are common in all cultures. Cultural changes, such as those produced by the civil rights movement of the 1960s, or the recently popularized push to decrease our carbon footprint, eat sustainable foods, and otherwise "go green," often come about in the ongoing attempt to resolve the contradictions in core orientations. Such changes may bring about new contradictions, and even produce a backlash.

Another result may be the formation of deviant or **countercultures**; these entail alternative lifestyles for those who cannot conform to or actively oppose widely accepted social norms. Because biomedicine is a part of the dominant culture in the United States, those alternative medical movements that reject the biomedical approach, such as Christian Science, exist, at least in terms of medical systems, as countercultures.

While countercultures emerge in opposition to the dominant culture, a **subculture** is generally considered a group within a larger group: a subgroup (meaning a subset, with no implication of inferiority) that lives within the general norms of a dominant group while preserving, to an extent, a unique lifestyle. The differences between cultures and subcultures may be based on political affiliations, socialization experiences, language, ethnicity, age, religion, occupation, health status such as disability, class, gender, and so on.

The various health care professions, for instance, form subcultures. When a person decides to become a doctor, for example, he or she will learn not only a new vocabulary, but also a new way of seeing that goes with that vocabulary. As a Harvard medical student explains, "In a sense we are learning a whole new world. . . . because learning new names for things is to learn new things about them. If you know the name of every tree you look at trees differently. Otherwise they're just trees" (Good and Good 1993, 98).

Regarding patients, another student said, " 'At first you are very aware that you are dealing with another person. Now I just don't think about that any more. You just do the routine' " (Good and Good 1993, 101). Added another, " 'I've had some real perception changes of people. . . . More and more, I can't help but think of us as machines' " (96). Becoming a doctor—or an acupuncturist, or nurse, or *Vodun* (sometimes spelled Voodoo) priestess, or any kind of health worker— is a process of acculturation as much as the result of long hours of hard work and study.

Subcultural groups and their members may be **bicultural**, functioning equally within their traditional milieu and the dominant culture; they also may hold to their own traditions while rejecting many of the dominant ones. Various groups may have become **acculturated**, having given up most of the traits of their original cultures and adopted those of the dominant group to a greater degree in some areas than in others. For example, they may reject the biomedical explanation of disease and its modes of treatment while fully accepting the dietary habits and patterns of dress of the dominant culture.

The United States is full of acculturating—and acculturated— people. However, **enculturation** (cultural socialization from birth) is such a powerful process that health crises often lead even the most highly acculturated people to return to their original cultural patterns. Seriously sick or injured people may also return to their native language and require a translator when brought in for care. It is therefore extremely important that the health provider have an appreciation of the various cultures and cultural nuances of the people served.

Is Culture All?

Despite the foregoing, behavior is not determined solely by culture, or any other one factor. A mental framework holding that one force determines how we think and behave is called **determinism**. Environmental determinism, for instance, posits that we are as we are due to the climate or environment of the geographic area we inhabit. Biological determinism holds that biology or genetic factors are key.

Biological factors surely do play a role in determining some dimensions of human lifeways. Genetic research, for example, is revealing a multiplicity of data regarding various populations' odds for contracting various diseases. However, genetic factors do not act alone to determine outcomes. Gene expression can be influenced by environment, as the emerging field of epigenetics has revealed. For instance, some genes related to obesity are turned on and off by environmental exposures to chemicals (Weinhold 2006). Our environments are, of course, in many ways culturally determined; we are the ones who pollute them. Further, much biological determinism is in actuality thinly disguised racism.

The case of erroneous arguments that IQ (a measure of intelligence) is determined by race is an example of such. Biased findings indicating that whites are intellectually superior to other groups are used to justify white oppression of nonwhites as biologically determined, or natural. But cross-cultural data shows that the intelligence measured by IQ testing is shaped by class and culture, not by race (see Fraser 1995).

This is easily seen in data from a study of children's intelligence published nearly 40 years ago. The study (Cole 1975, as cited in Nunley 1995) tested children's grasp of the idea of conservation, "the idea that when you pour all the water from a short glass into a tall glass, the same amount of water is still present, or if you take a fat ball of clay and roll it into a long narrow string of clay, the same amount of clay is there" (Nunley 1995, 76). The study was carried out with children of potters in Mexico and children in a West African fishing village. When water was used, the fishing village children did better, but when clay was used, they were outscored by the potters' children.

The majority of research shows that racial differences in IQ mask inequalities linked to poverty and limited life chances (Nisbett 2005). Further, differences have little significance in terms of actual intelligence; they measure only a narrow (and culturally determined) type of cognitive achievement (Gross 1992, 222–23).

In the **nature versus nurture** debate, nature, or biology, is pitted against nurture, or culture, as the explanation for the human condition. In reality, neither is true; both positions are too extreme and too simplistic. Real human thought and action is the outcome of a complex interplay of nature and nurture—of cultural, biological, social, psychological, economic, and political variables, all themselves historically contingent. In part because culture forms the framework within which social, economic, political, and other such changes take place, in anthropology as well as in sociology, culture is key.

ETHNOCENTRICTY, MEDICOCENTRICITY, AND CULTURAL RELATIVISM

CULTURE BLINDNESS

Culture from either the anthropological or sociological perspective can be seen as a measure of human flexibility. Its study reveals the amazing diversity of ways and means of meeting human needs under all sorts of conditions. Culture is both an abstraction and a blueprint or guide for social analysis as well as something enacted and negotiated. By studying the various elements of culture, we can begin to understand different social groups, the cultural contexts in which they function, and the links between cultural context, healing institutions, and human behavior related to illness and help seeking.

Loudell Snow has studied African American medical practices for many years. Snow describes the case of John and Eva Thompson (pseudonyms). The Thompsons had brought their baby, Patty, to the pediatrics clinic for her first immunization. Snow, affiliated with the clinic in her capacity as an anthropologist, sat in on the consultation (1993, 95).

The doctor administered the shot and then asked if there were any questions, and the parents had none. However, as soon as the doctor had left the room, Mrs. Thompson turned to Snow and asked if she had ever heard of using catnip tea for colic. As Snow tells it, "I replied that I knew it was a popular remedy in the neighborhood—but that I had always wondered how people knew how strong to make it. Mrs. Thompson's response was, 'Why it *says* right on the box!'" Mrs. Thompson also told Snow that adding a bit of honey made the tea taste better to the infant, and she and her husband told Snow a few other things about their medical traditions as well as their medical history—things that the attending physician was never told (1993, 95–96; italics in original).

When Snow shared with the physician the important medical history information that the woman and her husband had provided, she was annoyed. "'I don't know why these people always tell *you* everything'" (1993, 96; Snow's italics), she said to Snow. "It does seem obvious," Snow reflects, "that the initial question about catnip tea was a test: Mrs. Thompson clearly knew about catnip tea for colic, exactly how to prepare it, and, in fact, was already using it. Had I responded in a negative fashion she probably would not have gone on" (97). The Thompsons were worried about the possibility of being negatively judged for their practices—of being the victims of ethnocentrism. Their story is two decades old now but remains iconic; and such worries (and strategies) are of course not limited to African Americans. Many have observed similar scenarios (e.g., Prussing et al. 2004).

Ethnocentrism involves using one's own standards, values, and beliefs to make judgments about someone else. The standards against which others are measured are understood to be superior, true, or morally correct, while those being evaluated and not "measuring up" are inferior or wrong. Ethnocentrism can be observed in all types of cultural, social, and even personal evaluations when we condemn the customs, ideas, behavior, values, and beliefs of someone else when they are different from our own.

Ethnocentrism can also be observed regarding the tenets of science and medicine, which as noted may be considered natural or "correct" and therefore outside of cultural considerations. This attitude has been termed **medicocentrism** (Pfifferling 1981, 197). A medicocentric view focuses on disease, identified through signs and symptoms, and not on the patient or the patient's perception of a problem. The medicocentric physician uses a **reductionist** model, trying to make a diagnosis by narrowing (or reducing) the problem to medically explained phenomena (**disease**). But the patient may attempt to expand and relate the problem to his or her own perceptions and experiences, such as inability to carry out daily functions, symptom recognition and interpretation, misfortune, and discomfort (**illness**).

Physicians, as products of their own cultures, as well as of their medical training and occupational subculture, may exhibit both ethnocentric and medicocentric attitudes, which compounds the problem of bias. Let us say, for example, that Ms. Jones, a working-class woman has come to see Dr. Smith, who has confirmed her suspicion that she is pregnant. Dr. Smith also finds that she is malnourished and requires a great deal of prenatal care. Ms. Jones happens to be unmarried. Dr. Smith does not think that unmarried women should have babies. He lectures Ms. Jones on the use of birth control and pointedly mentions the option of tubal ligation (a form of sterilization). He writes a prescription and recommends certain foods and vitamins, as well as time off work and daily walks, without considering that

Ms. Jones cannot afford the food, supplements, and prescriptions, or that she must continue working in order to pay the rent, or that her neighborhood is not conducive to strolls. The probability of her following through on all of his recommendations is extremely low (DiMatteo and DiNicola 1982, Chapter 5).

CULTURAL RELATIVISM

The concept of **cultural relativism** requires that we objectively consider actions, beliefs, values, and norms within their own cultural contexts in order to understand them. It demands a situated understanding of what people do and because of this it generally clarifies the "why" through an appeal to cultural context. Cultural relativism asks what functions various cultural elements serve within that cultural context and how they are sustained, not whether they are "good" or "bad" by external standards. Cultural elements are deemed not better, not worse, just different.

One example of this is body modification (e.g., tattooing, scarification, penile circumcision) practiced in some cultures in initiating boys into manhood. Different cultures promote different forms of modification (Burton 2001). In cultural context, the modifications mark the body as mature, ensuring certain social rights and obligations to their bearers, and are painful—but not life threatening. Therefore, they may be acceptable within the framework of cultural relativism.

Cultural relativism presents some difficulties, however, when cultural beliefs and practices are harmful or based on cultural biases that in turn cause harm. They may even have legal implications from the perspective of the dominant culture. Furthermore, acts of torture, terrorism, oppression, persecution, poverty, suffering, and disease in any society have repercussions around the globe. In short, cultural relativism does not imply that practices must be accepted; *cultural relativism does not require moral relativism* as well. And yet, when we practice cultural relativism we are sometimes pushed to adopt—or assumed to hold—a morally relativist position as well. Because of this, just where to draw the line in determining whether cultural relativism is a helpful part of the health care process can be a difficult question.

Take, for example, female genital surgery or modification, sometimes referred to as female genital mutilation, or FGM, which is practiced in a number of countries. The hood of the clitoris, the clitoris itself, or the clitoris as well as both the inner and outer labia are removed. The latter form of the operation, which is most common in the Sudan and Nubian Egypt, is called infibulation: "The two sides of the wound [are] then stitched together, leaving a small pinhole opening for the drop by drop passage of urine and menstrual blood" (Gordon 1991, 5).

The practice of FGM is based on an ideal image of the female body as lacking certain parts of or all external genitalia (as opposed to male bodies, on which external genitalia are expected), and the belief that by removal of these body parts females will not become sexually active or desirous, will remain virgins until marriage, and will be faithful afterward. Moreover, the clitoris is considered as "dirty," and the female is not fit for marriage until it has been removed and she is "clean" (e.g., Gordon 1991, 9). One name for female genital operations is *tahara*, meaning purity. While in cultures that value FGM, females without it are stigmatized and denied most social options, FGM is excruciatingly painful, nontherapeutic, and medically can be very dangerous due to infection and ensuing debilitation.

FGM gained increasing recognition in the early 1990s as globalization brought populations that practice FGM in contact with those that do not. Some immigrant groups have been said to be importing specialists to perform the ritual. Physicians in the United States who have seen the results of FGM have strongly condemned it (e.g., Toubia 1994).

Intercultural contact produces diffusion, adaptation, innovation, and change, hopefully for the better. The human rights position can easily be defended on the basis of the fact that all cultures are in constant flux; that is, even so-called tradition changes and, therefore, traditional practices need not be cast as sacrosanct. Traditions may become outmoded and impractical. But all peoples have certain rights by virtue of being human. Perhaps surprisingly, it was not until relatively recently that this stance was encoded in the International Bill of Human Rights (United Nations 1978).

HUMAN SIMILARITY, HUMAN DIVERSITY: THE MULTICULTURAL SOCIETY

In the past, the United States promoted assimilation, and many of its citizens—old, new, and aspiring—boasted of its status as a great melting pot. Corporations even offered classes to immigrant workers regarding "American" ways of behaving, and some penalized workers who did not assimilate fast or well enough. However, the values and promises of equality produced a rising demand in the later twentieth century for respectful treatment of, as well as pride in, cultural diversity. Indeed, in the 1960s the United States experienced a cultural backlash against racism and discrimination as well as a push for numerous and long-overdue social and legal changes.

Many of the United States' core values are values to which all cultural groups can relate, such as opportunities for a better life for one's children (Glazer 1994). The uniquely American creed includes common values of dignity, equality, inalienable rights, freedom, justice, and opportunity for all human beings (Myrdal 1944). The fact remains that the United States is and always has been a magnet for immigrants and, accordingly, a multicultural nation. Indeed, the most recent available three-year estimates of the U.S. Census Bureau show that about 12.5 percent of the nation's population is foreign-born and 19.6 percent speak a language other than English at home (U.S. Census Bureau 2009). Demographic predictions are that "multiculturalization" will continue and increase. By 2050, it is likely that the United States will have no single majority group (Smelser, Wilson, and Mitchell 2001, 1). In medicine, as in other realms, there is a need both for cultural knowledge and consideration, as well as for finding the balance between our cultural differences and those commonalities that unite us all.

CULTURE, HEALTH, AND ILLNESS

Culture affects our perceptions and experiences of health and illness in many ways, and these perceptions and experiences change as culture changes. Health problems of any group can be affected by a multitude of cultural variables, some very basic. How we learn to subsist may depend upon the available foodstuffs and our abilities to adapt and utilize our environment. Custom and habit may produce sanitary or unsanitary living conditions. For example, the diets of migratory hunter-gatherer people were dependent upon the environment and climate. Because they moved from place to place, they never stayed around one area long enough for their own waste to bring about health problems.

The rise of agriculture and then urbanization created all manner of environmental health hazards in poor sanitation, overcrowding, starvation, and new vectors or conduits for disease. Technology solved some of these problems primarily in developed countries—and then created others, including pollution, more lethal weaponry, and toxic chemicals. Social stratification, too—including between as well as within societies—has led to health disparities, for instance in regard to who has access to clean water and therefore who is more vulnerable to waterborne illnesses like cholera.

Other cultural variables are conceptual. For instance, we have different ideas about health itself. A sociological study in France identified four ways of defining what health is: People saw health as either (1) the absence of illness, (2) a resource, (3) a controllable product of the individual, or (4) a "collective heritage for which society is responsible" (Pierret 1995 [1983], 195). These understandings seemed to be linked to social class or people's position within in a society.

What is illness to one person, or one culture, may be no problem to another, and vice versa. For example, in some cultures, what we in the United States call mental illness is not only *not* classified as illness, but is interpreted as favor from God in allowing an individual to understand or see what others cannot. Among the Navajo, for whom the prevalence of congenital hip disease is relatively high, treatment is simply not seen as necessary. Although it can eventually be painful, the condition is not seen as significant; resultant limping carries no stigma for the Navajo whereas it does for the mainstream American (Adair, Deuschle, and Barnett 1988 [1972], 206–7).

Ideas about the visible signs of health also differ; for example, many mainstream U.S. women strive for thinness while in impoverished Jamaica, a plump female body is much more appealing (Sobo 1994). The people of Fiji also like fat bodies, as these signify a wealth of social connections and financial resources and thus, "health" (Becker 1994). While in some cultures fatness is increasingly devalued due to the rise in diabetes seen in tandem with changes in diet and activity level that have meant individuals once merely plump are now obese, the long-standing equation between size and health has been harder to shake in areas where famine is still a likely hardship.

Cultures differ too on ideas of treatment for common health problems, and on preventive measures. To keep fit, a mainstream white American might go for a daily walk or join a health club to work out, while an African American might, in addition or as an alternate, take a laxative purge in the spring and several other times throughout the year (Snow 1993; cf. Smith 2001). A Native American might attend a "sweat lodge" ceremony, in order to purify and renew the spirit.

Health problems can be attributed to pathogens, accidents, or physical degeneration; they also can be attributed to supernatural means or relationships that do not meet idealized cultural standards, and they may be treated accordingly. In many cultures, health problems index social problems, as we will see. And they can entail not only physical symptoms, but behavioral or emotional problems as well. The subsequent chapters contain many examples of cultural influence in all areas of illness, disease, sickness, and healing.

FOR DISCUSSION

1. In what way are you a member of a culture or subculture(s)? Identify some of the customs that characterize the groups to which you belong.

2. Identify some instances of ethnocentrism that you have witnessed or heard about. What are some examples of ethnocentrism in health care?

3. Define cultural relativism and provide and discuss some instances in which cultural relativism might or might not be an appropriate part of health care provision.

CHAPTER 2

The Health-Related Consequences of Social Structure

GOAL: Understand how the social structure influences our positions and interactions with regard to our health, illness, and care seeking and delivery.

GOAL: Appreciate the related significance of the specific structural elements of family, ethnicity, social class, and gender in our health, illness, and care seeking and delivery.

Much of the tension in the clinical encounter . . . does not derive from the existence of diverse health subcultures, nor is it due to a failure in medical education to instill an appreciation of folk models of health and illness; rather, it is a reproduction of larger class, racial, and gender conflicts in the broader society.

(Singer, 1995, 85)

All interactions take place within complex social settings. A focus on beliefs and behavior (as expressed in healer-patient relationships), definitions and perceptions of health and illness, and decisions on whether or not to seek care and from whom has too often resulted in a neglect of the social-structural factors that influence those behaviors and interactions. In other words, while we may be interested to know how healers make their diagnoses or how people in different cultures decide whether they are well or ill (topics we examine in Chapter 4), knowing cultural rules is not enough. A consideration of social structure can tell us a great deal more about why people act the way they do. After defining what social structure entails, this chapter explores its ramifications for health and for health care delivery.

Just as each society has a culture or cultures to guide its members, each society also has a **social structure**. This refers to the organized patterns of relationships between individuals and groups within a society, which order their behavior in a predictable fashion and influence their interactions. Like culture, social structure can be seen as a **social construction**: as the product of social and power relations with complex histories and that are not fixed, but subject to change.

Culture supports, calls for, explains, and sometimes even masks structural arrangements involving kin, class, and gender, so that such arrangements are perpetuated. For example, the cultural value that health care should be available to every citizen may mask the reality that the structure of medical care delivery is not set up for such provision. If the system is not seen as requiring change, efforts to change it will likely fail.

Similarly, social, political, and economic structures support and make essential certain cultural ideals or forms. Laws concerning the acceptable makeup of the family, for example, support cultural norms concerning marriage (e.g., that it be monogamous). In this chapter, we begin to explore the interdependence between social structure and cultural expectations by examining concepts of family, ethnicity, gender, and social class.

THE FAMILY: A CULTURAL UNIVERSAL

All societies are divided in some way along the lines of **kinship**, which defines who is related to whom and in what way. Rules of descent and family structure vary across cultures, as does the importance of kinship. But all individuals belong to families of some kind.

Everyone who descends from the same line of ancestors belongs to the same **lineage**. In a unilineal system, a person is related by blood only to one parent's lineage. For example, the Navajo, a Native American group, are **matrilineal**. Therefore, a Navajo child belongs only to her mother's lineage. She is not related to her father's siblings' children as cousins in the same way as a British or Anglo-American girl would be. Those cousins are members of a different lineage. Ideas about relatedness have implications for medical record keeping and affect people's notions of what runs in the family.

Domestic Units

The domestic group most typically referred to by the term "family" in the United States is the **nuclear family**, which consists of a married mother (female) and father (male) and their unmarried children, living together. The marriage is considered **monogamous** and is, according to the ideal, sanctioned by U.S. law, which prohibits more than one spouse at a time.

A **blended family** is formed when people previously married with children get divorced, marry new partners, and then have more children together. There are also single-parent families, childless families, and gay families where the couple is of the same sex. The **extended family** consists of one of the aforementioned family units plus one or more grandparents, or may include an offspring's children, aunts and uncles, or other relatives.

Although nuclear, blended, and extended family units all, ideally, center around **conjugal** pairs (sexual partnerships), many families entail no such couples. That families without conjugal pairs are seen as aberrant is reflected in the terminology used to describe them, such as the "broken home" or even "dysfunctional" family. These terms imply that there is something wrong with a family in which there is a single parent. But single-parent families are aberrant only from the vantage point of a culture that idealizes a dual parenting arrangement and certain restrictive sexual arrangements. While in the United States the nuclear form is seen as the preferred family arrangement, it is actualized in fewer than one in four U.S. households (CensusScope n.d.).

A **household** generally involves a group of people who share living space at a given point in time, and who usually are—but need not be—kin. One person can also constitute a household. Household members sleep in the same complex and generally share food. A household is essentially an economic unit; it jointly produces goods or pools money and purchases commodities like power, water, and food.

People may belong to more than one household. In the United States, disadvantaged children's clinic records often contain multiple addresses, identify several different household heads, and list several different last names for members of any one household. Children may spend the day with one household and sleep in another. Household memberships change as different friends and relatives come and go in response to the changing events in their lives. As Carole Stack noted so many years ago in her now-classic study of kinship networks among impoverished black families, this represents a strategy for survival under harsh circumstances (Stack 1974).

FICTIVE KIN

A common American cultural variation of the family involves **fictive kin,** or people who are talked about and treated like kin with the full knowledge that they are not really related. Fictive kin may take responsibility for such things as protection, education, and health care of people who are not truly kin to them. Such flexibility is often seen among, for instance, Americans of African or Caribbean heritage. Urban black children with multiple caretakers tend to be less fearful about and friendlier toward strangers than their white counterparts, who seem to suffer more separation anxiety as a result of a rigid caretaking ideal in which a child can have only one mother figure (Snow 1993, 234).

Sometimes, fictive kinship entails ritual action and formal behavioral specifications. For example, many people of Mexican heritage (and Roman Catholics of other origins) practice *compadrazgo*, or godparenthood: Parents invite men and women to act as coparents when a child is expected and then born. The godparents are responsible for helping out, adopting, or fostering the child should anything happen to the parents. Pediatricians and clinicians working with populations that practice *compadrazgo* should be aware that sometimes they will need to deal with up to four coparents of one little patient, or that a culturally legitimate (if not legally sanctioned) adoption has taken place.

Family can thus be more usefully defined by function rather than structure. The family's functions, like structures, may vary, but are generally related to support, whether moral, emotional, physical, financial, social, or psychological. Functions may include protection, socialization, regulation of sexual behavior, affection and companionship, and provision of social status. They may also include reproduction, which contributes to human survival, or material and economic production, which also has benefits for survival. An often forgotten but essential function is the delivery of health care.

IN SICKNESS AND IN HEALTH

In many societies, the household or family delivers much of the health care, serving as the "hidden health care system" (Freund and

McGuire 1995, 174). The family functions as a support system and as a cost containment mechanism when, as a unit, its function has been disrupted by the illness or dysfunction of one or more members.

Even in a large-scale complex society, the patient who seeks health care is not afflicted solely as an individual but as part of a family unit; the entire group may be affected by his or her ill health. So, treating the patient also involves treating the family. Knowledge about various patterns of family structures and the need for family involvement is, therefore, essential for effective health care delivery in a multicultural society.

In biomedicine, treatment centers on the individual body. This is despite the fact that as long as 30 years ago studies had demonstrated a positive correlation between poor health outcomes and the level of stress in a home (as measured by such things as unemployment, communication problems, having a member with a chronic illness, a recent experience of divorce, death, or desertion, etc.). For example, Schmidt's early review of the literature found that high household stress correlated with a steady increase in streptococcal acquisition, illness, and a rise in antibodies. High stress also was related to increased risk of stroke, angina or chest pain, and concern with one's own and one's children's somatic (physical) symptoms. Pregnant women with high stress and low levels of social support had a pregnancy complication rate of over 90 percent (1978, 305–10).

Schmidt also found that when one's spouse had a disease, one's own somatic symptoms were likely to increase. And certain chronic diseases appeared in both spouses at a rate that was significantly higher than might be explained by chance (1978, 309). There were links between spousal death and the death of the remaining spouse from a number of causes including tuberculosis, hypertensive heart disease, influenza, and pneumonia (306). Likewise, divorce has long been known as unhealthy because of the stress it entails in certain contexts. Where divorce is not condoned, or when only one party seeks it, stress is heightened.

Further, good communication between clinicians and family members, and good family relations, have also been known for a long time to correlate with good rehabilitative progress. Compliance with clinician's recommendations also is better among patients with support from family members. For example, Schmidt (1978) reported that family empathy and support was shown to increase compliance in alcoholism treatment, to hasten the recovery process in stroke victims, and to elicit good response in patients with severe orthopedic disabilities.

On the basis of his review, Schmidt argued that there was "a definite advantage" in taking the family as the unit of medical care (1978, 303). This remains the case (Sobo 2003). Thus, in patient diagnoses, health care providers should be aware of the possible effects of life events, particularly those related to the whole family, as well as the family's role in day-to-day health maintenance and production, and make appropriate referrals for treatment.

WOMEN'S CONTRIBUTION TO HEALTH CARE

Speaking of the family as a care unit implies that all members of the family are involved in the caring, when they are not. "Family" is actually a code word for "women," used when discussing care at home (Ward 1993, 20).

Despite ideals of gender equality in the United States, women are still seen as nurturing caregivers and therefore are held responsible for health-related household tasks. Women bear the principal burden of care delivery for injuries or **acute** illnesses with sudden onsets as well as for the **chronic** and long-term problems of disabled and elderly family members. The responsibility falls most heavily on low-income women, often ethnic minorities, who have traditions of large families and of caring for their disabled and elderly (Ward 1993).

The household production of health involves more than just curing and caring; it also entails the daily round of cleaning, cooking, and child-minding activities. Women also bear the brunt of these jobs, often working a double day, both outside and inside the home. Their own health can suffer accordingly (Ward 1993).

Family involvement in care of family members, however, can also help offset the problem of rising health costs. For example, family members can be taught to give injections or monitor diets, or be empowered to help with other forms of therapy in order to avoid costly hospitalizations and to reduce emergency room visits due to avoidable at-home complications after initial hospital stays. Increasingly, strategies to include and educate families in at-home care procedures are included in formalized hospital discharge protocols. In light of this, efforts to better gauge family preferences for involvement are increasing (e.g., Sobo 2004).

Many people have the idea that home care is free, saving the rest of society a heavy financial burden. But this does not take into account wages lost by those who temporarily leave the workforce, losses in opportunity for job promotions and pension benefits, and the cost in health and well-being of the caregiver, who then may become unwell and poor and must in turn rely on her kin for unpaid care (Ward 1993). Additional costs involve various sacrifices the family as a whole must make in terms of its own financial needs, including saving for children's education and parents' retirement. However, much more research is needed on the actual burdens and consequences of caregiving.

CARE AND THE CHANGING FAMILY

In the past, without technology to keep us alive for longer periods of time and under more severe circumstances, the length of time spent caring for disabled or frail elderly family members was limited. Further, changes in family structure wrought by industrialization and modernization have produced care-related difficulties. First, the size of the average household has declined, mostly due to a rise in single-person and single-parent households (Chadwick and Heaton 1992). Indeed, by the year 2000, only 23.6 percent of all U.S. households comprised a married couple living with children under the age of 18. Just over 7 percent were female-headed households; just over 2 percent were male-headed. Over one-quarter (28.1 percent) contained married couples with no children, and the rest (39.1 percent) were variously made up of singles (25.8 percent), roommates (6.1 percent), or adults living with adult children (7.1 percent) (CensusScope n.d.).

Importantly, nearly one-third of households headed by single women are poor (National Poverty Center 2006). Besides the decrease in husbands' support for wives, we have seen an increase in dual-career or -employment patterns. Many people are involved in care of other family members to the limits of their abilities. Assessments of family context are crucial in determining the burdens entailed in, and abilities of individual families to be a part of, caregiving while still remaining a viable family unit that can function socially and financially.

DOMESTIC VIOLENCE

A health hazard that cuts across cultures and social classes is domestic violence, which produces physical, mental, and emotional damage, and is generally (but not always) carried out against women and children (see Durose et al. 2005). Domestic violence is not a new problem, of course, but it has generally been kept secret within the family.

Given the general value that mainstream U.S. culture places on family autonomy, health professionals may still look for easy answers (e.g., a fall down the stairs) or ignore the problem. They may also feel helpless and fall back on the claim that their role is to heal visible wounds, not to intervene in situations beyond their expertise (Gayford 1994).

Many factors are involved in domestic violence, including alcohol and drug use, psychiatric disorders, personality problems, jealousy, and various types of stress, social isolation, lack of coping skills, economic and other stresses, and social learning (Gayford 1994). Once taught to recognize the signs of domestic violence, health care professionals are in a good position, if trust of the victim can be gained, to recommend counseling, psychological treatment, and in extreme cases, referral to a shelter (in the case of children, many states have laws requiring reporting of suspected violence). Health care professionals can promote the idea that domestic violence is no one's right, is not acceptable, and need not be tolerated.

PROVIDING CARE FOR THE FAMILY

A number of possible solutions to the general problem of family care for the disabled, elderly, or chronically ill have been considered, but in general intervening here does not fit the cultural view held by mainstream U.S. society in regard to family autonomy. Solutions summarized by D. Ward (1993, 24–25) include superior adult day-care centers; new types of housing designed for different types of families; institutionally based care in the home with families providing some assistance; community and public service centers offering health clinics, day care for elders and preschool children, and community lunch facilities; housing partnerships; shared spaces like apartments linked to community health workers' offices; and services for cleaning and meal preparation. Such possibilities have been tried in some locales, but they continue to face strong opposition because our society assumes that the problem of chronic care is the responsibility of, and will be addressed by, families (mostly women—and some men). These assumptions in part supported drastic cost cuts made in conjunction with the economic crisis of the late 2000s, to some of such programs that did exist. Denial of assistance was and is further fueled by the aforementioned assumption that at home such care is free, with no cost to society.

Perhaps the message for all caregivers, both professional and lay, is to take time to understand the power and limitations of the family, whatever the culture and however structured, in health, illness, and recovery or in simply maximizing quality of life for everyone concerned. Family structure and environment are essential elements in a patient's diagnosis, treatment, recovery, or rehabilitation.

Fuller and Toon (1988), in discussing the various family structures related to minority populations, include two propositions for dealing with families with structures different from one's own, and those still stand today. First, there is the need for at least an intellectual understanding of any given family structure and its dynamic—of how it functions. Second, there must be an emotional acceptance that different types of family structure may operate with the same degree of success (or failure) as the structure accepted in the practitioner's own culture (69).

Families are composed of different kinship ties and relationships, but they are still families with strengths and problems. Some families have more resources than others, some have strong beliefs relating to health, illness and caregiving, but all are subject to general social and economic conditions that affect abilities to respond to health and illness, whatever the cultural or ethnic origin.

Like family structures, ethnic, class, and gender identities also affect and influence the perceptions, relationships, and responses of both health care givers and receivers, as well as the general structure of caregiving institutions. They are also linked into the global political economic system, such that habits—and health problems—that seem to be local or individual may actually have been engendered by larger sociopolitical considerations.

THE CONCEPT OF ETHNICITY

Ethnicity is tied to notions of shared origins and shared culture. In the United States, ethnicity is reflected in the classifications of Mexican American, German American, and Polish American, for example. Even without an explicit national or continental qualifier, all Americans are members of one or another **ethnic group**. White middle-class American ethnicity, for example, can be identified through commonly preferred television shows, modes of dress, and viewpoints, including views on who qualifies as a member of their group.

Ethnic groups form when one group of people expresses an identity different from those with whom they share borders. These borders can be national, but they also can have to do with the distribution of power in a society and factors on which this power is based, such as skin color, religion, income, language, and country of origin. The ethnicity "Native American," for example, emerged when America was colonized. Aspects of the divergent identities of the many existing tribes merged when groups who previously might have been at odds came together in a united effort to resist colonization and cultural annihilation.

Ethnic identities are constantly being invented and modified. Further, they are not permanently fixed to the individual, although they may be ascribed on the basis of visual criteria, such as skin color, which cannot be easily changed—although its cultural significance can vary. And specific practices entailed in an ethnicity can be forgotten, or adopted not only by whole groups but also by individuals (such as in giving oneself a new name or in forgetting one's native language). In this way people can, under certain circumstances, merge with or separate from a specific ethnic group.

An individual may have many ethnic identities, especially in a multicultural setting. And these can, in certain situations, be used selectively: Individuals can shift back and forth between identities as they see fit. For example, a provider or patient may use English in the clinic setting but another language at home. One may eat certain foods when lunching with colleagues at work or in a clinic waiting room but different foods at home. Adopting a role specific to another ethnic group does not imply hypocrisy; as different contexts call forth different dimensions of the self, one may simply be exhibiting the self that is most pertinent in a given situation (Goffman 1959). Or, of course, one can be simply trying to "pass," to get by, or to avoid problems such as being discriminated against, or subjected to harassment, physical violence, or even killed.

Minority Status and Health

Members of certain groups may have very little input into the social system that governs them. This **minority status** reflects their lack of opportunity, access, and participation, rather than number. Minority status, in turn, affects health status.

For example, like other migrant workers, Mexican migrant workers travel continually as crops are ready for harvest. Their health care is thus fragmented, with no follow-up or continuity. Further, migrant workers usually work through the heat of the day with little or no time to rest or cool off. Employers sometimes fail to supply accessible toilets;

with open fields and no shelter, people sometimes wait the entire day to urinate or defecate, creating various intestinal and kidney ailments. Water is sometimes not supplied for hand washing and so, after picking crops dusted with insecticide, workers ingest toxic substances with lunches (see Baer 1996; Bollini and Siem 1995).

Black Americans have also, as a group, suffered poorer health than white Americans: "Poor health is a structural feature of Black existence" (Quimby 1992, 161). In other words, poverty, powerlessness, and the racism that these conditions are tied to severely limits the health care options open to black people while greatly expanding their health challenges. For example, infant mortality rates are twice as high for black people as for white ones (MacDorman and Matthews 2008). Infants that do survive are challenged in their fight for survival: A study of mortality rates in New York City in the 1980s revealed that men in Bangladesh, an impoverished and underdeveloped nation, are more likely to reach the age of 65 than black men in Harlem (McCord and Freeman 1990, as cited in Snow 1993). This finding is still cited widely today (e.g., California Newsreel 2008c). However, there is some good news: The black-white life expectancy gap has declined slightly in recent years, narrowing for men from 8.44 years in 1993 to 6.33 years in 2003, and for women from 5.59 to 4.54 years (Harper et al. 2007).

One reason for the gap's persistence is that racism is pervasive in the health care system (see Funkhouser and Moser 1990; Barr 2008). As Hutchinson (1993) notes, it exhibits itself in cursory physical examinations, deficient bed assignments, delayed admissions, and assumptions of noncompliance; further, racism often overlaps with class-based discrimination against the poor, and it influences the adoption, implementation, and administration of health policies that limit certain aspects of the lives of lower-income people. As Hutchinson observes, "Access to health care in the USA is usually dependent on ability to pay for it" (1993, 10–11), and of course many African Americans are poor. Navarro notes that the problems are rooted in the social structure, and that "it is unlikely that by concentrating solely on race differentials we will ever be able to understand why the health indicators of our minorities are getting worse" (1994, 494).

The gap also is fueled by the interaction between biology and culture. Racism can, in fact, result in a heightened amount of stress in those who experience it. Chronic stress writes itself into the body, altering for example heart function and insulin-related processes. The bodies of people under chronic stress are therefore more prone to diseases such as hypertension and diabetes. They also are more prone to premature labor, which contributes greatly to infant mortality rates. Hypertension, diabetes, and infant mortality—long known to occur at higher rates among black people than among white people in the United States—are therefore in many ways the result of our culture's racism. In an interesting twist, these conditions may be exacerbated by the myth that racism is no longer a problem: This myth intensifies the stress that accompanies racist treatment because it raises expectations for nonracist treatment to begin with as well as implying that racism will not be seen by others as having been real. (See Wyatt et al. 2003; see also Mays, Cochran, and Barnes 2007; California Newsreel 2008a, 2008b.)

Self-Perceived Compliance versus Noncompliance

All things being equal (which of course they are not), some blame for health inequity lies in simple miscommunication. For example, Mrs. Hibbert, an African American, was told by her doctor never to eat pork, so she gave it up. However, Mrs. Hibbert never extended her understanding of pork to include pork fat. She served Snow a tasty lunch of greens and cornbread, prepared with liberal portions of bacon grease. Even as she cooked, she talked about her doctor's instructions, and how much she missed ham (Snow 1993, 142–43).

Likewise, a man diagnosed with high blood pressure stopped taking his pills. When he went in for his monthly exam, the staff was shocked to see that his pressure was elevated. They asked about his medication, and he freely reported not taking it. He reminded the staff that a blood test he had been given last time indicated that he should stop the medication. This caused much confusion, for the only blood test the man had had was a routine blood count. But then he reminded them that the doctor had said his count was a little low. The man took this to mean that his blood pressure medication had thinned his blood and needed to be discontinued until balance was restored (Snow 1993, 134).

Misunderstandings, such as those reported, are responsible for a good deal of what clinicians patronizingly call "noncompliance." However, some patients do not want to take medicines prescribed and do not intend to do so. This is the case across the board, for all ethnic groups, albeit for sometimes different reasons. Among the black population, this can be because patients see doctors' medicines as too strong, or too chemical, or addictive (Snow 1993, 271). Many prefer their own home remedies to those that doctors might prescribe. They may go to the doctor for diagnoses, not for treatment. Others go to make sure that their own treatments are doing the job or that their health conditions are under control.

ETHNICITY AND MISTRUST

Sometimes, people do not adhere to clinic medication recommendations because they fear being poisoned. This is particularly so for black Americans. Many link black fears about the intentions of white health professionals directly to their knowledge of the historic and exploitive Tuskegee Syphilis Study. The study, which began in the prepenicillin year of 1932, involved documenting the natural course of untreated syphilis in about 400 poor black men. The men were manipulated into participating in the study by promises of free medical treatment and financial incentives.

The study was originally planned as **cross-sectional**: It was to involve a single, time-limited effort in which researchers would examine men in various stages of the disease to ascertain the damage that it would theoretically do over time to a (male) body. The original recruits did receive the then-standard heavy-metals therapy (which involved mercury and arsenicals). But then authorities decided to turn the study into a long-term **longitudinal** effort, and cases were to be observed until "end point": autopsy. The men did not receive antibiotic therapy when it became available in the 1940s (Edgar 1992; Jones 1992).

Exposure of the study by the media in 1972 led to its termination and, ultimately, to the passage of the National Research Act in 1974. The act mandated that proposals for all federally funded research involving human subjects be reviewed by boards that may reject any proposals deemed unethical or scientifically misguided.

In any case, the Tuskegee research—research funded by the U.S. government's Public Health Service—involved letting people die. Knowledge of this fuels rumors. For example, people often assume that the Tuskegee participants were intentionally infected with syphilis. While such assumptions may be false, the historic facts of the study cannot be denied. The feelings and knowledge that lead people who do hear about the Tuskegee study to draw erroneous conclusions often stem from life experiences. And perceptions of racism and maltreatment are validated by the knowledge of the study's existence, causing people who learn about it to cling to it as "a symbol of their mistreatment by the medical establishment, a metaphor for deceit, conspiracy, malpractice, and neglect, if not outright racial genocide" (Jones 1992, 38). The personal experience of racism and a legacy of negative encounters with the public health system fuel the misgivings that many minorities have about health care workers' motives and intents.

ETHNICITY AND THE BODY

Some minority health problems do appear to be genetically linked, such as Tay-Sachs disease in some Semitic peoples, sickle-cell anemia in some blacks and certain Asians, and diabetes in some Native and Mexican Americans. Genes certainly do matter. However, recent research in the emerging field of **epigenetics** reveals that environmentally induced biochemical reactions that occur around or on top of our genes can actually control their expression, turning them off or on, meaning that certain genetically linked disease states (although of course not all) may in fact, instead of being inevitable, be triggered by humanly created environmental conditions, such as diet or toxic exposures (Gillman 2005; Weinhold 2006). For instance, the social structure contributes greatly to various susceptibilities and risks, as through poverty, and connections between stress and conditions such as hypertension (see California Newsreel 2008a, 2008b; Dressler 1990; *Economist* 2009; Wyatt et al. 2003; Mays, Cochran, and Barnes 2007).

Assumptions regarding genetically linked differences extend, to a certain degree, to visual characteristics such as skin color, facial features, and hair texture. While these traits will differ more according to one's specific geographic background than to one's purported race, members of minority groups have been known to be pressed into having plastic surgery so that their features are made more "mainstream."

Often, operations are justified as being beneficial to health. This is the case with upper-eyelid surgery by which some East Asian people effect a more Anglo appearance. It can be rationalized as a biomedically necessary procedure to remove what some doctors call "excess fat" (Kaw 1993, 81), and to fix eyes that are "too narrow" (82). Some women have been told by their doctors "that it was 'normal' for them to feel dissatisfied with the way they looked" (81).

Minority peoples also have been made to feel badly about overall body shape and size, or ways of styling the hair that do not conform to mainstream U.S. standards. For example, some African Americans who wear dreadlocks or beaded and braided hairstyles have been ordered by employers to alter their hairstyles. Hygiene concerns may be voiced to rationalize such orders, although dreadlocked or beaded braided hair is much less likely to be shed than hair in a straight or loose white style. And people whose body ideal is plumper than the thin mainstream cultural ideal have been pressured to lose weight, even though we now know that the ideal weights used by insurance companies to indicate health risks change periodically, and may be underestimated, and that some people are naturally heavier than (and just as healthy as) others. While obesity has generally been found to be unhealthy, the cultural perception, including that of biomedicine, of what constitutes obesity is variable (Mumford 1983, 148–49). For instance, Americans' ideals for weight increased between 1990 and 2007: women's average ideal weight went from 129 to 138; men's, from 171 to 178 (Newport 2007).

THE EFFECTS OF POVERTY AND SOCIAL CLASS

SOCIOECONOMIC STATUS

Conditions that may at first glance appear to be correlated with ethnicity or other variables may actually be due to relative poverty and, thus, to social class. Social class in the United States is generally measured by a combination of income, occupational prestige, and educational variables. Together, these index socioeconomic status, which can generally be expressed as upper-, middle- or lower-class membership.

The United States is characterized as having an **open class system**, which ideally means that there is a great deal of **social mobility** between class categories or levels, and that social position is earned, or **achieved**. This structure is the opposite of a closed system, where social position is **ascribed**, or assigned at birth and in which there is no social mobility. In actuality, most systems—ours included—lie somewhere in between. Various ascribed characteristics, such as ethnicity and gender, may also affect our opportunities for achieving higher social positions.

The dominant ideal cultural value of equal opportunity in the United States reflects the myth that "anyone can make it in this society if they really want to." Real values limiting social mobility through discrimination by ethnicity, sex, age, religion, and socioeconomic status are revealed in **structural barriers**. These barriers may consist of poor educational facilities and preparation, denial of employment in certain fields, or few or no promotions to positions of power, and consistently low wages and lack of benefits for certain groups. Poor health or disability also can block social mobility.

SICKNESS AND POVERTY

Poor people are definitely sicker than the well-off, largely because of poverty conditions. Their **life chances** (meaning opportunities for acquiring favorable life experiences) are accordingly affected through loss of opportunities for advancement of personal and social goals. Barriers to mobility may also be created for other family members, who must care for those who are ill.

The ill or disabled may be seen as lacking skills that they actually do possess, so they face discrimination much in the same way that members of ethnic minority groups do. Moreover, much poor health and disability is seen as resulting from individual behavior. This ignores the role of social structure as a causal factor.

While poverty causes much sickness, in some cases it is also true that sickness causes poverty. For example, a person who becomes ill with a chronic condition may be denied employment and insurance and may expend all his or her resources and savings to the poverty level.

ETHNICITY, GENDER, AND FINANCIAL POWER

Like the ill and disabled, ethnic minorities and women are at a distinct disadvantage regarding financial resources or control. A good part of this disadvantage can be attributed to structural factors such as the types of jobs available to these populations and the prevailing wage scales. As the hourly wage fails to respond to the cost of living, people find themselves working two or three jobs just to meet basic needs or perhaps not meeting them at all. Types of jobs held disproportionately by members of minority groups and women include unskilled labor and service jobs that pay very little, offer few benefits, and are vulnerable to periodic layoffs.

Although risk factors are multiple and complex, studies consistently show higher rates of **mortality** (death), **morbidity** (disease), and disability among the lower classes (see Isaacs and Schroeder 2004; Rose and Hatzenbuehler 2009; Pappas et al. 1993, 103–9). Explanations have included all the concomitants of poverty—poor housing, more exposure to pathogens, unemployment, poor education, less access to health care, discrimination, strenuous and dangerous working conditions, poor sanitation, and high stress. Additional factors would include higher risks for violence, high levels of drug and alcohol use, and high-risk sexual behaviors, which can also be related to social structural pressure.

ACCESS AND UTILIZATION

Present patterns indicate that low-income groups are the highest utilizers of health care in hospital settings, where services may be overcrowded, uncoordinated, hurried, and impersonal. Conversely, as income level increases, so do visits to office-based physicians (Centers for Disease Control [CDC], 2008b).

Relative to need, the poor may still underutilize services. Although inadequate insurance coverage is a factor, so is a lack of emphasis on preventive care and denial of illness due to the more pressing needs of survival, such as the need for food and shelter. Poor people generally receive treatment for symptoms at home rather than preventive care and thus may be sicker when they do seek official medical help. In general, cultural perceptions and variations tend to be less important than economic necessity in the decision to seek care. For example, Haitian peasants hold complex ideas regarding the link between sorcery and tuberculosis, and one might be tempted therefore to assume that this explains underutilization. However, cultural ideas often serve to ease the pain of lack of access rather than promoting it. When a group of Haitians were afforded supported access to treatments previously out of reach, they were quite happy to accept them, with high rates of compliance too (Farmer 2005).

The factor that best explains low utilization in relation to need is what early on Dutton (1978) called the "systems barrier." This involves location, availability of and transportation to facilities, time needed for consultation, and the negative experience of poor patient-physician or patient-provider relationships. Moreover, as more recent studies have shown, the skill to gain access to begin with, and the ability to navigate the system once in, are crucial (e.g., Sobo, Seid, and Gelhard 2006).

Of course, the poor are more likely to be uninsured or to receive Medicaid funds, which many doctors do not accept, so the places of treatment for the poor are more likely to be limited to hospital outpatient clinics and emergency rooms. Access to medical care, however, still falls far short of explaining class differentials in health status and life expectancy. Several studies done in Great Britain, where health care is available to all through the National Health System, show that the provision of health care to poor populations did not affect the levels of disease and illness in that population; nor did it eliminate the difference in health status between social classes (Hollingsworth 1981; Reid 1989; Marmot, Shipley, and Rose 1984; Whitehead 1990).

Patterns also emerge from U.S. data indicating that morbidity differentials by class are much larger than by race (Isaacs and Schroeder 2004; National Center for Health Statistics [NCHS] 1988). Both blacks and whites in lower–socioeconomic status groups have higher rates of illness than blacks and whites at higher income levels.

Syme and Berkman (1994) point to the existence of gradients in which the lower the social class, the greater the mortality and morbidity rates (also see Barr 2008). The differential includes virtually all disease conditions. Syme and Berkman point out, "That so many different kinds of diseases are more frequent in lower class groupings directs attention to generalized susceptibility to disease and to generalized compromises of disease defense systems" (31). This suggests again the connection of mind-body, social conditions, coping mechanisms, and physical, psychological, and cultural vulnerability; it confirms the need to focus on how the stress of poverty and discrimination may compromise the immune system, making one more vulnerable as stress increases. Learning to cope may help alleviate stress, thereby lowering the risk of illness (Benson with Klipper, 2000).

However, there is a danger that focusing on individual coping and the idea that teaching people to cope with their poverty or life changes will solve the problem. Simply blaming people for not coping—or for coping through the use of tobacco, alcohol, narcotics, or drugs and violence—only relieves pressure on the social system to change. And with no real change in the expanding structural environment of poverty, there will be no *real* change in the health of the poor.

For health care providers, empathy for low-income patients and an understanding of the effects of poverty can go a long way toward making such patients more comfortable and satisfied, opening up avenues for care seeking and health education. It is also essential for those providing care to examine their own attitudes, beliefs, and motivations relating to racism. Because there are so many variables that may be contributing to illness, it is vital to try to discern something more about patients' lives and environments than simply their socioeconomic status classification (see Chapter 7 regarding how). It is also useful to have some knowledge of support systems, agencies, and contacts where some help may be found, including referral services, social workers, food supplement programs, support groups, or other public services and agencies.

Although we have emphasized poverty's effects on health and health-related behavior here, the effects of economic advantage should not be forgotten. They are implicit in statistics on the health of the poor. The health of those with economic means is the yardstick by which poverty's effects can be measured. Wealth confers power, and also affects attitudes toward health workers, as the following hospital case study shows.

The study further shows that the influence of social factors, such as class, rarely occur in isolation. The privilege that class buys the individual described next is augmented by the structure of gender relations that he draws on when dealing with the nurses assigned to him when treated in a U.S. hospital.

Hamid Sadeghi

[Hamid Sadeghi] was a twenty-five-year-old upper-class Iranian. . . . He was very uncooperative and refused to do anything for himself. He would ring for the nurses and demand, "You get here right now and do this." He would not, however, accept anything he had not specifically requested, including lunch trays and medication. He posted a sign on his door that read, "Do not enter without knocking, including the nurses." His attitude caused a great deal of resentment among the nurses. Why did he treat them this way?

When asked, Hamid responded, "This is the way it is done." Finally, one of the nurses who had an Iranian brother-in-law recognized the behavior and explained. Traditionally, Iranian men are dominant over Iranian women. They give orders to women, not take them. Furthermore, as a member of the upper class, Hamid was probably used to giving orders to servants. He was not purposely being difficult but merely acting in his customary manner. (Galaniti 1991, 23)

Mr. Sadeghi's wealth gave him the upper hand in most of his social relations, and he expressed his power even in the hospital setting. His wealth-backed expressions of power toward female nurses was fortified by the structure of gender relations in his culture.

GENDER ISSUES

GENDER OR SEX?

While **gender** differences have to do with ideas about what it is to be masculine or feminine, **sex** has to do with biological differences between males and females relating to reproductive functions. Sex differences are, for the most part, genetically determined. Babies are sexed according to the type of external genitalia they are born with.

This method of categorizing individuals generally works fairly well. But in some cases, internal biological signals become mixed, resulting, for example, in individuals who exhibit the external sexual characteristics of both sexes. Some are born internally male and externally female, or the reverse. The genitalia are not a foolproof indicator of genetic sex. Of course, the idea that one's genetic sex is somehow one's true sex is itself culture-bound. So are the ways in which male-female biological differences are perceived. Where biomedicine today sees differences between the male and female reproductive systems, other cultures' versions of biology see similarities. So even sex, which is a biological category, is not necessarily an unarguable "natural" fact.

Notwithstanding, the technical concept of sex generally differentiates us into male or female. Gender is manifest in socially and culturally constructed masculine and feminine roles and expectations for behavior. Notions of gender, or of masculinity and femininity, generally entail the assumption that certain abilities, traits, skills, and capacities fitted to particular tasks and activities are specific to each sex. Having said that, there are theorists who argue that in some cultures a third gender actually exists; others see third gender as simply a cross between masculine and feminine—despite the fact that some qualities noted in this merging or crossing are not inherent in either of the original categories crossed (see Roscoe 1992).

Gender is generally ascribed in a way that squares with perceived sex: Males are generally brought up to act and think in a (culturally defined) masculine fashion, and females in a (culturally defined) feminine one. Gender socialization affects one's life chances as well as one's behavior and thoughts. For instance, certain educational, occupational, and even health opportunities are reserved for one gender or the other.

GENDER AND POWER

While many gender-linked associations are culturally specific, others are found cross-culturally and can be explained as based in fundamental differences between male and female physiology. For example, because of their biological childbearing role and because they can breastfeed, women cross-culturally are generally highly involved in caring for infants. Some theorists have argued that it is precisely because women are so busy with child care that men have been able to hold the power in many societies (e.g., Sacks 1974).

In such societies, which are called **patriarchal**, men are in control. The more patriarchal a society is, the less important women, and all that is associated with them, are deemed. This devaluation serves an ideological function, supporting male domination. Negative stereotypes of women also may stem from "procreation envy" (Bettelheim 1962, after Freud). In other words, men may feel jealous that women can have babies and they cannot. One way that men can gain the upper hand is by trivializing women's procreative power. So, for example, menstruation and birth become associated with nastiness and uncleanliness; menstruating women are banned from certain places or tasks. Further, sensibilities and skills associated with the female gender are devalued.

In addition to trivializing female functions, men may appropriate women's procreative power. They can do this in various ways. Bettleheim describes certain male-only religious rituals in which men perform sacrifices and other acts designed to ensure fecundity. If women's fertility depends on men's rituals, then men are the true masters of childbirth (see also Burton 2005 for a summary of examples). Medicalization is another way by which men control women's procreative power; we discuss this process in Chapter 5.

Early European stereotypes of women as breeders and nurturers and men as property owners and controllers were part of a patriarchal and patrilineal system of inheritance (Turner 1995). They have survived in various forms in modern societies—even within the medical institutions. This is reflected in medical textbooks (Martin 1990) and in the occupational division of labor, as for doctors and nurses (and within the doctoring category some specialties are seen as more masculine and others as less so; see, for instance, Cassell 1998). Even in the face of contradictory evidence, old gender stereotypes remain strong, due to people's beliefs that gender roles are "natural" (biologically determined) or divinely ordained. Ultimately, the strength of these stereotypes may derive from political expediency: They support vested interests in maintaining economic control of resources and the current distribution of power.

NATURE OR NURTURE?

For years people have debated to what degree gender roles represent something "natural" or something cultural—or something in between, or of an entirely different order. Back in the late 1920s, anthropologist Margaret Mead (1963 [1928]) described typical behaviors of each gender in three different cultures in New Guinea—the Mundugumor, the Arapesh, and the Tchambuli. When compared to American behavioral expectations for men and women, Mead found considerable differences.

In two of these cultures, there was little gender role differentiation; one might say that these were one-gender cultures. Both male and female roles in the Arapesh were what would be considered feminine by U.S. standards—both were equally maternal, gentle, and home loving. The Mundugumor would have been considered masculine—both males and females were hostile and fierce, seeming to care little for their children.

In the third culture, the Tchambuli, the role expectations were the reverse of those found in the United States. The women were solid, practical, and powerful providers who hunted and fished. The males were emotional, concerned with their appearance, enjoyed decorating their homes, and pursued the arts (Mead 1963 [1928]).

If females are by definition indeed passive, overly emotional, non-intellectual, weak, submissive, and nurturing, then all females in all societies should exhibit these characteristics. The same would be true for all males being stoic, rational, active, intellectual, and so on. Mead found that this was not the case. Biology, in other words, is not destiny.

SEXUALITY

Sex has to do with biology, gender with culture, and **sexuality** with the expression of erotic desire. In the United States and similar cultures, ideas about gender include the assumption that to be masculine is to desire sex with women and to be feminine is to desire sex with men. These ideas, which are not universal (Davis and Whitten 1987, 81, 83), support the current American family-based norm of one mother (female) and one father (male) and are sanctioned by law and religion. Therefore, bisexual and homosexual identity and behavior (i.e., sexual attraction to and interaction with people of either sex or the same sex, respectively) may be seen not only as nonnormative but as immoral and a threat to the entire society (Abelove 1994). Homosexual and bisexual people are thus subject to a great deal of hostility, stigma, and discrimination in the general society. This bias can run over into the clinical setting. It is imperative, however, for clinical effectiveness, to leave personal opinions regarding sexuality outside the office door—especially when assumptions about what is "normal" are themselves culturally constructed.

Kinsey and colleagues' famous 1948 study of sexuality showed that in a population of 5,000 white American males, 37 percent reported at least one homosexual experience to orgasm as adults (Kinsey, Pomeroy, and Martin 1948). This calls into question the definition of homosexuality in men. How many experiences—if any—must one have to be labeled homosexual? Many individuals who have repeated same-sex liaisons do not identify themselves as homosexual or gay and many who have no sex at all do identify as such. Further, many people who would be labeled, by either themselves or society, as homosexual actually may frequently engage in heterosexual intercourse (Gatter 1995).

Homosexual behavior is practiced by people of all cultures and is found in all classes, occupations, and professions, including medicine. Because of oppression, many gay men and lesbians remain "in the closet," unwilling to allow their sexual orientations to become known.

Homosexual people face real barriers to quality health care because their sexual health needs are often ignored or denied. Health clinics rarely display posters or pamphlets depicting same-sex couples, but heterosexual pairs are frequently used. Women seeking pap smears or other regular gynecological screening may simply be assumed to be heterosexually active; questions such as "what type of birth control are you using?" can effectively stifle candid discussion of homosexuality (or asexuality or abstinence for that matter). Homophobia—whether a clinician's or a patient's—certainly stifles candid discussions of HIV/AIDS-related risk, necessary not only for harm reduction education but also for appropriate HIV screening; thus, it can hamper access to care (Sobo et al. 2008).

GENDER IN MEDICINE: TEXTBOOK EXAMPLES

Because attitudes and ideas regarding gender expectations are perpetuated through the process of socialization, healers within a society are subject to them like everyone else. Our biases are clearly shown in the language we use to talk about biology. Immune cells are described in various medical publications as making up an "infantry" of "mobile regiments," "snipers," "soldiers," "bodyguards," and even "killer cells" that "shoot lethal proteins" at enemy invaders (Martin 1990, 412). In part due to the historically male makeup of our armed forces and the metaphor of battle, the imagery evoked is perceived as purely masculine. This becomes more apparent when the hierarchy of immune system cells is examined.

As Martin explains, the so-called lower cells—the ones that engulf dying enemies and clear up debris—are generally described in feminine terms. The process of forming a pouch for engulfing or eating debris is called "invagination," and certain medical texts actually refer to the pouch as "vaginal" (1990, 416). Heroic male killer cells shoot enemies and female drudges clean up the mess. While there might be many other ways of talking about what takes place (e.g., as a food chain), and there is no scientific reason to attribute gender or sex to cells that have neither, gender imagery is predominant in this discourse, and gender stereotypes are reinforced each time that we use this discourse in teaching or talking about the immune system.

Gender stereotypes permeate all levels of the health care system, and can be found in the interactions between doctors and patients as well as in medical textbooks and medical laboratories. For example, because masculinity is constructed as nonemotional, many men do not show emotions when they feel them. Others may not even feel them at all; sometimes, suppressed emotion ends up being expressed in sickness.

Because women are ranked lower than men in the gender hierarchy, gendered health treatment generally has a more severe and negative impact on them. For example, physician Robert Wilson (1966) advocated massive doses of estrogen for women at menopause in order to keep them "feminine" (by which he meant youthful). For Dr. Wilson, the female sex was defined by their ability to menstruate and their culturally defined physical beauty, the loss of which rendered them "neuters." Menopause was considered, by Wilson, a "disease condition" expected to produce dangerous physical and psychological symptoms even though the number of menopausal women actually suffering any bothersome symptoms at all is estimated to be only around 20 to 30 percent (Corea 1977, 266).

Wilson was not an exception and the views he espoused remain pervasive. Fifteen years after he wrote, sociologists Diana Scully and Pauline Bart (1979) reviewed 27 modern gynecological textbooks and found the prevailing stereotypes of women expressed in recommendations for diagnosis and treatment. Women were seen as fulfilled only by reproducing, mothering, and looking after their husbands. They were expected to be passive and subservient, and health for women was defined as marriage and childbearing, while deviance from this norm was defined as disease producing. This has changed somewhat in the United States but very little: Martin, for instance, noted that menopause was imaged as a factory shutdown in books she examined (1987). In 2005, a National Institutes of Health panel announced that menopause should not be considered a disease. They were concerned that medicalization can lead to the use of risky, questionable, and unnecessary treatments.

And what of Wilson's estrogen cure? The National Women's Health Network reports that "feminine forever" has been replaced with "young at heart," in which estrogen is promoted as prevention for heart disease, based on a recent Women's Health Initiative study. Disconcertingly, this is even though the WHI data showed that taking estrogen gave "no protection against heart attacks and slightly increased the risk of other types of cardiovascular disease, including blood clots and strokes" (National Women's Health Network 2007).

The idea that women's bodies (or minds) are defective has been reflected in the fact that women have long received more prescriptions for medications than men, even for similar problems and conditions (see Corea 1977, 91–95). Use rates have increased for both groups over time, but the difference has increased, too: Between 1988–1994 and 2001–2004, the proportion of men using at least one prescription in the past month rose from an average of 32.7 to 41.6 percent; for women it went from 45.0 to 51.5 percent (NCHS 2009, Table 98).

The disparities in terms of surgical intervention are also notable regarding women. The rate of hysterectomies (surgical removals of the uterus, or womb) in America is consistently oddly high, especially when compared to other industrialized countries (Eagan 1994, 23; Payer 1996, 125; Keshavarz et al. 2002). Hysterectomy is the second most frequently performed surgery on American women of reproductive age, second only to cesarean section (Keshavarz et al. 2002). Culture plays a strong part in biomedical decisions.

As with gynecological health, mental health has been defined according to adjustment to culturally constructed roles and expectations. For instance, in the 1960s, a group of psychologists, psychiatrists, and social workers were asked which traits characterize healthy, mature males, females, and (sex-unspecified) adults. They reported little difference in expectations for a mature, healthy, competent adult and a male. For a mentally healthy female, however, traits given were those that are considered (in our culture) as negative and even child-like: submissive, easily influenced, not adventurous, dependent, feelings easily hurt, excitable in a crisis, conceited, subjective, and disliking math and science. The mature man was a mature adult; a woman was expected to behave immaturely in order to be considered healthy and mature (Broverman et al. 1970). As the study authors state:

> Acceptance of an adjustment notion of health, then, places women in the conflictual position of having to decide whether to exhibit those positive characteristics considered desirable for men and adults, and thus have their "femininity" questioned [or be labeled as maladjusted or even mentally unhealthy or ill] or to behave in the prescribed feminine manner, accept second-class adult status, and possibly live a lie to boot. (6)

An "adjustment" notion of either physical or mental health must, by definition, be related to the social structure and culture. Adjustment may mean conforming to a socially constructed ideal that supports a particular power structure in the society. Broverman and colleagues suggest, for example, that black persons who conformed or were "well-adjusted" to the stereotype of the pre-civil rights African American as passive, docile, childlike, and happy would be considered healthy, mature adults (1970, 6).

While much progress has been made against previous biases and beliefs, it often comes slowly and with social resistance. For example, homosexuality was removed from the American Psychiatric Association's list of mental disorders in 1973. However, it was not until 1992 that the World Health Organization removed it from the international list.

Diagnostic criteria thus reflect attitudes, beliefs, and values instilled in health professionals as they grow up. Enculturation leads to different labeling, diagnoses, and treatment of men and women. Because health care providers are expected to be the experts, their behaviors and actions, and ultimately social and medical policy, in turn support and perpetuate stereotypes. It is therefore necessary for the providers of health care to examine and correct for their own stereotypes and biases (see Chapter 7).

GENDER, MORBIDITY, AND MORTALITY

Male-female differences are not confined to differences in diagnostic standards. They infuse health status statistics as well. Women, for example, have higher rates of acute illness such as infectious, respiratory, and digestive problems not related to pregnancy. They also have higher rates of certain chronic, long-term conditions such as hypertension, anemia, colitis, migraine headaches, arthritis, and gallbladder problems. Men have higher rates of accidents and injuries, gout, emphysema, and coronary heart disease. Men also have higher rates of cancer in the youngest and oldest age categories, while women have higher rates between ages 20 and 55 (Cockerham 2010, 67). However, these statistics are affected by psychosocial and methodological factors.

For instance, while research using different measures and data sets found that women reported more mental and physical symptoms, there was no gender difference in self-assessed general health. Patterns of gender morbidity have been shown to vary considerably according to ethnicity, life stage, class, and age, as well as status of females (Arber and Thomas 2005). When generalizations are made regarding male-female mortality and morbidity and assumed to apply across the board, our full understanding of their underlying causal pathways is thwarted.

There are also male-female differences in patterns of health care utilization. Women use health services more often than men, even when maternity services are excluded. Although reasons for this pattern of care seeking are far from clear, some possibilities include the fact that women employed in lower-paying jobs lose less for time off, plus the fact that they are more aware of health status (especially when they have children), and receive more positive reinforcement for care seeking (Verbrugge 1990).

Men may be more stoic than women about pain or health problems. Women may place a higher value on health, and they may be more willing than males to admit to and acknowledge symptoms and attend to them as well as report them, which is consistent with role expectations (Weiss and Lonnquist 1994, 55–56).

Although on average women report more illness than men, in the United States they can expect to live about five years longer on average (Hoyert, Kung, and Smith 2005). This holds true across ethnic and socioeconomic groups. Part of the explanation for these differences clearly lies in expectations for gender behavior. Men are more vulnerable to death through violence and accidents than women are (Waldron 1994, 45, 49; Arber and Thomas 2005, 102). To be masculine in America, one takes risks: Men's heavier drinking, greater gun use, less safe driving patterns, and higher rates of smoking have significance for male mortality patterns (Waldron 1994, 49). Cross-culturally, more men than women smoke, and in the United States from one-quarter to three-fifths of the sex difference in mortality due to ischemic heart disease may be related to cigarette smoking (46). With more women in the workplace holding higher stress jobs and engaging in more risk-taking behavior, and with lower rates of smoking in men, we may see some of the differences evening out.

Other attempts to explain the differences in morbidity and mortality include biological or sex-linked differences, such as women's childbearing risks. Still, differing trends over time and their historical explanations confirm the heavy influence of social and behavioral factors. As Arber and Thomas state, "A gender analysis of health needs to be sensitive to the ways in which social, economic, and political factors affect gender roles and relationships, and the consequences of these for health" (2005, 108).

Women's experiences with cesarean sections neatly demonstrate the influence nonmedical factors have on treatment decisions. The cesarean operation was named for Julius Caesar, who was said to have been cut from his mother's womb. The operation itself, which constitutes "major surgery," has saved many lives and helped to reduce both maternal and infant mortality rates. But the increasingly inappropriate use of the operation for nonmedical reasons has become problematic.

In 1970, the rate of cesareans in the United States was around 5 percent. The figure leaped to 25 percent by 1988 (Eagan 1994); by 2006, nearly one-third (31.6%) of deliveries were cesarean, making the "C-section" the most common operating room procedure in U.S. hospitals. Concurrently, data indicate that cesarean births are associated with higher rates of rehospitalization and postpartum medical care use for new mothers. Further, worse outcomes for babies delivered this way have been noted (Russo, Wier, and Steiner 2009).

Today, privately insured women receive 34 percent of cesarean sections and uninsured women receive 25 percent. What this means is not clear, but it appears that those who have easier access to this surgery via insurance are opting more frequently to use it. In the 1990s, the leap in cesarean rates was interpreted against the advantages of the cesarean for the physician as well as the hospital, which included more predictable and convenient birth scheduling as well as a larger fee (Russo, Wier, and Steiner 2009). Today, however, scholars have become interested in women's reasons for opting for cesarean births, and these include scheduling convenience and avoidance of childbirth pain. They also include fear over infant outcomes, which has been linked to a cultural construction of vaginal birth as dangerous and a preference for technocratic or surgical control in that case (Hewer, Boschma, and Hall 2009; Davis-Floyd 2003). Some women also have expressed concerns over vaginal structure—concerns related to internalized expectations regarding women's sexual role.

Paradoxically, not only have women been inappropriately over-medicated and overtreated (by whosoever's choice), they have also been undermedicated and undertreated—and not just for lack of access. Women have, for instance, been accused of a tendency to "overreact" and to imagine various symptoms. One study found that men's reported symptoms (including chest pain, fatigue, headaches, and dizziness) were taken more seriously, generating thorough work-ups in every case. These symptoms were often dismissed when reported by women (Eagan 1994, 23; Rieker and Bird, 2000).

In now-classic work, Irving Zola (1983), when reviewing some previous research on problems of ethnicity in doctor-patient communications, realized that when the males in the population had reported symptoms for which there was no organic cause identified, they were given "non-judgmental diagnoses," while for females the same types of complaints were noted as either "psychological or of no clinical significance, depending on ethnic group." Zola also observed that all the examining physicians were white males (134).

Today, more women are entering the medical field, which may be a force for change. Women account for half of all medical school applicants, and half of all graduates. They comprise 42 percent of all residents and fellows, and 32 percent of all medical school faculty members (Magrane and Lang 2006). Both medical care providers and patients may be greatly affected by gender, power differentials in the workforce, and the systems and institutions within which they work and receive care.

MICRO, MACRO, AND GLOBAL SYSTEMS

Macro-level or institutional, social-structural arrangements determine how, where, what, to whom, and by whom care is delivered (e.g., on the basis of ethnicity, class, or gender); that is, they affect health-related experiences at the **micro** or personal, immediate, and interactive level, which involves the web of interpersonal relationships.

Global systems entail structural arrangements that incorporate not just one society but others as well. Biomedicine, as practiced in various countries, comprises a global system of care. As the world grows smaller and nations and peoples become more interdependent, more and more links connect the micro and macro levels with global systems and issues. Macro-level and global arrangements can have great impacts on health at the personal micro and community levels— impacts often far greater than those that culture per se may have (Baer et al. 1986; Singer 1995). The connections between and among all three levels of organization may be noted in the following case.

Hector Velez, a Mexican immigrant to America diagnosed with cancer, seemingly "made a habit of not showing up for scheduled doctor's appointments and then arriving unexpectedly" (Galanti 1991, 29). Some might argue that Mr. Velez was, in keeping with his culture, acting on a "present time orientation, which is inconsistent with clock time . . . Someone with a strong present time orientation would tend to get involved in the activity of the moment and not think about the time necessary to get somewhere at a particular hour" (30). Others might explain Mr. Velez's behavior as conditioned by the institutional arrangements for health care in his native country: Many clinics in Central America (as well as other parts of the world) do not offer appointments to patients but allow people to call in at their convenience and wait to be seen.

However, both explanations ignore the larger social-structural factors conspiring against Mr. Velez and other people in the lowest economic classes: "Many poor people have difficulty getting time off from work to make an appointment. Public transportation is not always reliable. For the poor, life is often a matter of moment-to-moment survival. Advance planning is a luxury that can often be enjoyed only by those with money" (Galanti 1991, 30). And money Mr. Velez did not have. Nor did he have a car, or a phone, or even indoor plumbing. As a social worker investigating his case found out,

> His home was a broken-down toolshed behind some shacks, which he rented for $75 a month. His shower was a garden hose and his bathroom a neighborhood gas station. He slept on a soiled mattress on the floor and kept his clothes in orange crates that doubled as tables and chairs. He had spent the last three years working as a farm laborer and had recently begun collecting recyclable cans and newspapers to support himself.
>
> (Galanti 1991, 30)

Clearly, more than a present time orientation was behind Mr. Velez's appointment-related behavior; his poverty was key although his personal behavior was what was reproached. The policies and priorities of macro structures such as government, which lead to or do not address problems of poverty, provision of education, adequate food supplies, and employment, also underlie this behavior.

Further, Mr. Velez's predicament was related to the global level of international politics and economic conditions in Mexico. International borrowing, debt loads, discriminatory policies, corruption, rising and falling international markets, international political and economic priorities and interests at home and abroad all may have affected Mr. Velez's needs.

Mr. Velez's case demonstrates how many macro level forces can come together to support particular health-related actions and outcomes. When they do so in a way that limits an individual's control over their health outcomes, **structural violence** is at work. This violence is not quick, like a gunshot, but slow and steady, stemming as it does from historically given, economically driven arrangements (Galtung 1969). Class and caste systems are examples of structurally violent systems. Health inequities can result from the structural violence systematically inflicted on those occupying lower positions in the social structure.

SYNDEMICS

Mutually reinforcing epidemic health conditions that occur at the same time and contribute to an excess burden of disease in a given population also can be created when macro-level forces converge. These are called **syndemics**. Tuberculosis, malnutrition, and HIV/AIDS form a syndemic in certain populations. Found more commonly when people are living in poverty, they cluster together, reinforcing and exacerbating one another—as they are reinforced and exacerbated by the social structure. Building on the simple idea of comorbidity, the syndemic concept emphasizes the connection between conditions and the multiplier effect that one has on another (Singer 2009).

At the global level, the reality of potential catastrophe brought about by human processes, such as travel, modernization, war, and trade, becomes all too clear when we consider the simultaneous spread of such diseases as HIV/AIDS and tuberculosis. As the world grows smaller, we cannot escape the possibilities of a global medical disaster, precipitated by social and cultural means as populations come into contact with each other and disturb the ecology. The need, then, is for a cooperative approach that considers the social-structural factors that contribute to the dangers, and integrates the efforts of various systems to prevent disease and provide care and treatment.

Such an approach must also take into account the structural impact on diverse health needs that arise at different stages of life, such as in protecting children and caring for aging populations. The next chapter examines health from a life course perspective with the aim of generating an appreciation of yet another dimension of human diversity—and similarity.

FOR DISCUSSION

1. What are some of the ways in which social structure determines and influences various health problems in a population?

2. How do the various elements of the social structure help determine who gets sick and who gets care, and what kind of care they get? What significance does "blaming the victim" have in determining causal factors of disease? Which victims are more likely to be blamed?

3. How are cultural ideas used in support of structural barriers or facilitators to health care? How are they used to confuse the barriers to care, or even hide their existence in relation to family? To race/ethnic group? Social class? Gender?

4. How can health care clinicians incorporate broader knowledge of families, ethnicity, social class, and gender into more effective caregiving?

CHAPTER 3

Health and Illness Over the Life Course

GOAL: Identify the life course concept's usefulness and explore different perspectives on health and illness in the context of life stages.

GOAL: Achieve an awareness of the ways in which the stages of the life course are—and are not—culturally diverse, and how they relate to our health needs and perceptions.

Life cycle stages are often determined by biological events, but each is played out in a cultural context that defines and characterizes it.

(Ferraro, Trevathan, and Levy 1994, 160)

The life course provides an excellent framework to discuss and assess questions about differences in needs related to health, illness, and care. For example, this orientation allows us to ask: How are possibilities for health, illness, and responses to illness related to various cultural perceptions of being an adolescent or an adult, or to a society's attitudes and values regarding old age? How do cultural variations in the approach to birth and death relate to giving birth, being born, and dying? And how can socially situated awareness of the cultural context of life stages aid the health care provider as well as the recipient of care? We also can ask how events in one stage may affect another.

One of the difficulties in using a concept of life course is deciding where to draw lines dividing one stage from the next. Some studies break the life course down into chronological categories such as "birth to 1 year," "1 to 5 years," "5 to 10 years," and so forth. It is more useful here, however, to consider the culturally specific developmental categories of infancy, childhood, adolescence, adulthood, and old age.

While individuals in the same stages of the life course have much in common, such as their general biological development and capacities, the various roles they have experienced, and the perspective of the number of years they have lived and have yet to live, life stages are not delimited in exactly the same way cross-culturally. The culturally defined life stage of adulthood, for example, may begin earlier among certain groups (e.g., with first menses or at a certain age, say, 13) and later among others (e.g., when a bachelor's degree has been completed or employment first secured). Some of the life stage guidelines deemed important in one culture are deemed inconsequential in another; even the recognition of particular phases such as life stages can differ cross-culturally. For example, the time after death when one becomes an ancestor is not a life stage for the biomedical clinician, but it is for some Japanese Buddhists (LaFleur 1992).

Further, to conceive of events happening in stages implies delimited events rather than a life continuum, and that each designated stage has a norm. Anything outside the norm may be viewed as abnormal and thus subject to negative labeling and medical or social intervention. Relating to biomedical practice, Stein (quoted in Dossey 1991, 122) observed that "the physician may hide behind the metaphor of the 'stage' instead of confronting the unique person to whom these [stage labels] apply." And as Atchley (1994) notes, "The life course in reality is composed of a great many alternative routes to alternative destinations" (155); this makes normative sequences essentially unrealistic.

Still, various periods in the life course have specific ramifications in terms of our risks and possibilities of illness. In addition, our needs and vulnerabilities at any stage and how they are addressed can be and are mitigated, reduced, enhanced, and changed by cultural and structural factors and variables.

PREGNANCY AND CHILDBIRTH

Sociocultural context is relevant to us even before we are born. Various factors can affect the fetus in its development and potential, particularly the health and well-being of the mother. Her poverty, illness, isolation, exposure to toxic substances, stress and disease, accident and violence—all may affect the outcome of pregnancy for the baby, the mother, and the entire family.

The conditions and behavioral implications of poverty must be considered in any discussion of causes and preventive strategies. Women who have little education, cannot afford to adequately feed themselves and their families, cannot afford child care, are uninsured and have little or no access to health care (including prenatal care), and, if addicted to alcohol or drugs, have no access to substance abuse treatment programs, cannot be expected to remove their risks for or remedy the ills of poor birth outcomes by themselves. It is hoped that future research can tell us more about ways to break the cycle. We also need more research on the role of men, the influence of passive and active smoking, domestic violence, and substance abuse by the male on outcome of pregnancy.

PRENATAL CARE

Because most of these problems are preventable, various forms of intervention may be necessary and desirable to protect babies' and mothers' health and well-being. Therefore, the most important consideration before birth, and (structural issues for now aside) one that relates to education and cultural factors, is prenatal care. Education is an essential part of prenatal, as well as postnatal, care; and cultural sensitivity and awareness is a necessary part of any prenatal or postnatal care program. Such programs should also involve fathers when this can be done without alienating the target community. It should be recognized that in some cultural groups, especially where levels of sex segregation are high, the father is proscribed or effectively denied and excused from participation in certain activities involving pregnancy and birth.

Another cultural issue has to do with targeting care. One of the most basic and grave errors made in political as well as in social and medical discourse on prenatal care is the culturally influenced failure to consider mother-to-be and fetus as a unit. If mother and fetus are considered separately—which a culture valuing individualism may encourage if the fetus is seen as an individual—it is possible for an adversarial relationship to develop in which the question simply becomes one of whose rights prevail (Johnsen 1987), as in the U.S. abortion debate.

The issue of autonomy has arisen in numerous legal challenges regarding where to draw the line for maternal responsibility and fetal rights. For example, statutes have even allowed children to sue their mothers for behaviors or actions while pregnant that may have adversely affected the child's development prior to birth (Johnsen 1987).

Technological capabilities such as intrauterine surgery have raised questions as who is really the doctor's patient—the mother or the fetus. Such a question could arise only in a particular cultural context; here, gender power structures and technological ideals are at play (see Davis-Floyd 1992). If the mother refuses such surgery, even if due to the risks it may impose on her own health, is she guilty of potential harm to the fetus? Johnsen (1987) notes that women make countless decisions that create some minimal risk of harm, as in driving a car or even in wearing seat belts. Further, we do not force someone not pregnant to undergo a medical procedure for the good of another, even for a child. Fetal rights laws ignore the fact that the woman cannot walk away from the fetus to avoid legal restrictions and liabilities. Pregnancy thus presents a completely unique situation, both medically and legally.

Another example of how rights questions surface has to do with genetic testing for genetic or congenital disorders. Advanced prenatal diagnostic systems that can pinpoint the likelihood of a given condition (such as Down syndrome) have underwritten pregnancy terminations by parents who decide not to carry an "at risk" or prenatally diagnosed fetus to term. The implications of this are not yet clear. Quality of care for those born with diagnosed conditions may suffer due to the decrease in clinicians' experience serving children and families with these conditions. Stigmatization may increase in keeping with a constellation of ideas regarding prevention, parental responsibilities, and which lives are worth living (Sobo 2010).

The issues raised could take us far beyond the focus of this chapter. Nonetheless, the points considered are strongly related to medical decision making and cultural attitudes and values. It is always much easier to "blame the victim" than to recognize the relationship of social structure, including political values, economic barriers, and social pressures, as the root causes of many health and social problems.

THE CULTURE OF CHILDBIRTH

Childbirth everywhere is "treated and marked as a life crisis event and as such it entails a multitude of beliefs and rituals meant to help both mother and child and sometimes the entire family or community pass unharmed through this period of danger" (Jordan 1993, 3–4). However, while even in very early ethnographies accounts of birth rituals can be found, little was actually known about the female experience of pregnancy and childbirth or women's secret procreative knowledge until recently. This is because anthropology was for so long a bastion of men who could not, in most cultures, be present at birth, let alone participate in women's culture. So it was not until female anthropologists were able to observe and chronicle birthing practices and knowledge from the woman's perspective that much of our present information was gained (Romalis 1981, 9).

In 1978, Brigitte Jordan first proposed that birth, a "universal biological function," is embedded in a "culture-specific social matrix" (Jordan 1993, 48). This matrix entails many interactional aspects. The local conceptualization or cultural definition of birth, which will include ideas about who should do it, when, and why, is one feature; birth also features pain and pain management, preparation (including formal or informal education—or the expectation of no instruction at all), attendants and social support systems, a territory or place of action, and technologies or artifacts. Importantly, the latter can determine birth position as well as limit the participation of the birthing mother in her own delivery. Women cross-culturally give birth in a number of positions, the most effective of which harness the power of gravity to assist in the expulsion of the fetus. Often, someone behind the woman supports her laboring body. Sitting, squatting, kneeling, and standing are popular positions. In a recent study comparing position preferences, the supported squat was most popular by far. These women reported all around better birth experiences with easier pushing and less pain (Jordan 1993, 85).

Notwithstanding, and still today (see Davis-Floyd 2003), the American hospital delivery table is constructed such that the only possible way a woman can give birth is lying on her back, in what is called a lithotomy position. The tables have no foot end; women's feet are put up in stirrups. This position decreases the size of the pelvic outlet and puts undue pressure on a woman's pulmonary and cardiac systems, lowering oxygen supply to the fetus. Contractions are weaker and pushing is harder because gravity can be of no aid. Vaginal and perineal tearing are more likely, as is the need for pain medication and labor-inducing chemicals. Further, as there is no space on the delivery table for it, the attending physician is forced to cut the cord to the placenta immediately, which means that the infant does not receive about 25 percent of the blood that it would otherwise take in (Jordan 1993, 84, 86).

In addition to position, distribution of decision-making rights and the ownership of authoritative medical knowledge are key. For example, in America, where the birthing mother has, still today with few exceptions, neither total control over decisions nor authority, a woman desiring pain medication may have to "produce the appropriate display of pain experience" to convince the attendant of her need for relief. This "adds to the comparatively high level of noise and hysteria in American obstetric wards but must also provide powerful feedback to increase the subjective experience of pain" (Jordan 1993, 53). In Sweden, by contrast, where pain medication is available on request, "the atmosphere is one of quiet, intense concentration rather than vocal panic and despair" (53).

A huge diversity in birth customs and beliefs exists, although some universal themes and obvious symbols surround the event. These include the themes of human continuity and women's power to give life (or nature's power to do so). Some universally potent symbols related to and often referred to in birth ritual cross-culturally are blood, water, milky substances, snakes, rope or cord, and eggs. Blood refers to menses, life blood, and the actual bloodiness of childbirth; water refers to amniotic fluid and drinking water as well as water for irrigation; milky substances are associated with breast and genital secretions; snakes shed their old skins and have newly regenerated ones underneath, as well as resembling the penis and the umbilical cord, which is itself represented in rope or cord, also representative of family ties; eggs symbolize the continuity of life, rebirth, spring, and life potential (cf. Romalis 1981). More specific meanings will also be found in each culture, where local beliefs as well as environmental and historical conditions will lead members to particularize the connotations of each symbol.

In rural Jamaican tradition, in which heavy ritual action is generally not undertaken unless there are problems with a pregnancy, simple preventive steps in which simple symbolism is manipulated are the norm (Sobo 1993). For instance, a mother-to-be avoids stepping over ropes or vines, to keep the fetus from becoming entwined in its umbilical cord. She does not tip her head back too far when drinking to avoid suffocating the fetus. A mother's food cravings must be met or her child's body will be marked; however, too much of one food can affect fetal development. Similar practices have been recorded for many cultural groups.

Superficially "superstitious" practices may be based in common-sense understandings about fetal development and about the effect that actions in one realm may have on another. As long as such practices do no harm, they can support a patient's sense of well-being, and they should not be discouraged by health practitioners. In fact, by making a mother feel good about taking culturally recommended proactive measures, other prenatal care practices, such as those promoted by biomedicine, can be encouraged. The same holds true for postnatal practice. Supporting a Caribbean woman who wants to pin a piece of red cloth or ribbon on her newborn's vest to ward off evil can help build trust and encourage her in taking up biomedically effective health promotion practices.

Some birth rituals may include the provision of social and emotional support during labor and birth. Among the Maya in Yucatan, who give birth in their homes, along with the midwife and the woman's mother, the father-to-be is present to support his partner both physically (he sits behind her) and emotionally. It is important for him to witness her pain (Jordan 1993). In American hospitals, strangers are often the only witnesses, although increasingly fathers and other significant others do participate.

In some cultures the man participates in pregnancy itself, experiencing morning sickness and other symptoms. Pregnancy is, then, not a private individual condition but one that affects the parents together. The anthropological term for this is *couvade*. Couvade signifies and tightens conjugal bonds, and gives a man what Moore et al. call "cultural confirmation" (1980, 118) of paternity. Reproductive rituals ensure the well-being of all. They also help cement social ties and reinforce social structural arrangements (see also Browner 1983; Browner and Sargent 1996).

THE BIOMEDICAL VIEW

Biomedicine views pregnancy and especially childbirth as medical events. Through **medicalization** of childbirth, physicians (and so their patients) tend to define and treat the condition of pregnancy as abnormal—a condition that only they can manage.

While millions of babies are born successfully without intervention of physicians, biomedicine has enjoyed great success in reducing the maternal mortality rate (Friedman 1994, 3). Women died from complications of childbirth at high rates before surgical procedures, such as the use of the forceps, to remove fetal obstructions were invented. Before the germ theory became widely accepted, however, physician-attended births frequently ended with the mother's death from childbed fever, or puerperal sepsis, because doctors did not recognize the need for cleanliness.

Childbed fever had not been a widely recognized problem prior to the advent of hospitalization during birth. It was Austrian physician Ignaz Semmelweis who first noticed, in the 1840s, a link between unwashed hands and the disease. He saw that in his hospital, women attended by doctors had a rate of childbed fever five times that of those attended by midwives. Semmelweis ordered hand washing with disinfectant, and a dramatic decrease in the disease was seen (Jordan 1993, 51).

While hand washing was clearly necessary, Davis-Floyd writes that "the removal of birth to the hospital has resulted in a proliferation of rituals surrounding this natural physiological event more elaborate than any heretofore known in the 'primitive' world. These rituals, also known as 'standard procedures for normal birth' work to effectively convey the core values of American society" (2003, 1–2).

Such rituals have included shaving the pubic area, giving the birthing woman an enema, and prohibiting any food intake. While these procedures have been rationalized as promoting sanitation in the controlled birth arena, they actually can lead to higher rates of infection, for instance through nicks made during shaving. A lack of nourishment saps energy and subsequently lengthens labor as well as increasing the acidity of any vomit. Enemas, which can be very painful, decrease neither the likelihood of elimination during labor nor the incidence of fecal contamination (Davis-Floyd 2003, Chapter 3).

While shaving and enemas have mostly been left behind, many hospitals still limit dietary intake. And plenty of other ritual procedures remain. Some, such as attaching women to umbilicus-like intravenous (IV) drips and fetal monitors, limit their mobility and confine them to the lithotomy position, which can prolong labor and necessitate further medical intervention in a domino effect. IV glucose drips can even lower women's tolerance to pain, necessitating more medication (Davis-Floyd 2003, Chapter 3). Of late, this has not mattered much to a growing proportion of women: Sargent and Stark have investigated how the information imparted in childbirth classes, as well as the ways that it is imparted, can help reinforce women's preference for intervention. As a result, for example, many women interpret the "elimination of feeling by means of epidural anesthesia" as "the ultimate definition of control in delivery" (1989). We discussed this kind of thing in regard to medicalization in Chapter 2; here we would add that it supports claims of the growing internalization among

American women of what Davis-Floyd has termed the "technocratic model" for childbirth (2003, 46–48).

Beyond the patient experience itself, another way to understand American birth ritual is through an examination of the experiences of nurse midwives (Rothman 1994, 104–12). Nurses' training is well grounded in the biomedical model. When becoming midwives, however, nurses are exposed to anomalies that challenge biomedical knowledge of childbirth. The differences primarily involve medically defined stages of the birth process, each of which has a statistically, biomedically estimated norm of time allotted.

Hospital births are speeded up when a particular stage is seen as taking too long. Intervention may be justified biomedically, for example as minimizing danger and discomfort to mother and baby. However, the number of hospital deliveries to be processed in a given period of time is a prime factor in the decision to intervene. If a woman's body's birth timetable is too short or too long, the routine of the hospital is upset; deviations are unthinkable (Rothman 1994, 111).

Thus when nurse midwives witness healthy out-of-hospital births in women who do not conform to the biomedical timetable, they begin to challenge the biomedical model itself. The range of "normal" becomes much broader and individualized (Rothman 1994).

INFANCY

INFANT DEATH

Throughout history, surviving infancy has been a challenge. Indeed, the relatively high likelihood of infant death or mortality figures into many cultural practices such as delaying naming a child until a certain number of days have passed, or withholding membership in the family until certain other milestones have been reached (e.g., eruption of first tooth). Even today, and even in the United States, infant mortality remains a challenge. Leading causes of infant death in the United States include congenital anomalies (birth defects), disorders related to short gestation and low birth weight, and Sudden Infant Death Syndrome, commonly known by the acronym SIDS (Centers for Disease Control/National Center for Health Statistics [CDC/NCI] 2009). Again, all may be related to sociocultural factors (see Chapter 2).

While infant mortality rates have declined steadily here, hovering now at about 6.7 nationwide (CDC/NCI 2009), certain subpopulations remain more vulnerable than others. For instance, the rate for African American babies is twice as high. This is largely due to structural and related cultural factors. Notwithstanding, it means that the United States ranks 28th worldwide for infant mortality (27 nations have lower rates) (Office of Minority Health & Health Disparities 2007).

Why are the rates so inflated for African Americans? To begin, African Americans are more likely to be poor than members of many other groups in the United States (see Barr 2008, 134–68). However, there is more to infant mortality than poverty per se. While poverty is no doubt a contributing factor, so too is racism. As noted in Chapter 2, the perception of racist treatment increases one's measurable stress levels and this is correlated with low birth weight, among other things, and mortality and morbidity rates are higher among such infants. The implications of broader social reality—and the legacy of colonialism and slavery—are obvious here (California Newsreel 2008b; Dominguez 2008).

Modern social arrangements implicate themselves in other ways in infant death statistics. A problem possibly related to family structure and modern lifestyle, SIDS accounts for 7.9 percent of all U.S. infant deaths. SIDS is thought to be tied to genetics, maternal smoking and drug use, young age of mother, infections late in pregnancy, and parent-infant sleeping arrangements. The latter seems particularly important. (March of Dimes 2005).

Preferred sleeping arrangements vary from culture to culture, but historically, and cross-culturally, sleeping with others—including with babies—has been the norm. Under safe conditions (not including, for instance, when a cosleeping adult is intoxicated and may overlay and suffocate a baby), such arrangements are protective. Indeed, as James McKenna and Thomas McDade argue, research data "show that co-sleeping at least in the form of room sharing especially with an actively breast feeding mother saves lives" (2005, 134). Among other things, cosleeping infants receive breathing cues from cosleeping parents (139–40). The importance of this becomes clear when we recall that the infant's cardiopulmonary system is, like most other parts of the infant's body, still quite immature. It benefits from external stimulation. Cosleeping infants receive this throughout the night. They also tend to be placed automatically in a back-down, face-up position; this simply makes sense for breastfeeding and it happens also to be protective against SIDS. On their backs, infants sleep lighter and are more reactive to their environment (138).

Unfortunately, the benefits of safe cosleeping were lost to many when postwar cultural shifts in the United States led those who were able to give infants their own rooms as well as to bottle-feed them. Both practices signified new-found affluence, the desire for early individuation of the infant, and faith in "science." Today, however, despite rhetoric erroneously casting cosleeping as dangerous and immoral at best, the number of mothers practicing cosleeping for at least part of the night is back on the rise, at least in the United States, UK, Australia, and New Zealand (McKenna and McDade 2005, 135). The challenge here will be to enable those living in poverty to take advantage of the benefits of correctly practiced cosleeping, which currently are beyond reach for many due to unsafe sleeping surfaces and various other barriers created or catalyzed through impoverishment and marginalization.

IMMUNIZATION

Up until the early twentieth century, infectious disease was the major cause of death for children in all societies. The turnabout was related to the invention of a range of immunization techniques and products by which vaccinated children were protected from what were heretofore killer diseases such as polio and whooping cough. Uninoculated children—and the ethnic or class groups they mainly represented—were culturally transformed into public health threats.

Despite their potential benefits, present-day immunization efforts sometimes fall flat in the face of a growing public distrust of the medical and public health establishment. Wealthier, more educated, white people actually are more likely than others to refuse vaccinations (9.7 percent as opposed to2.8 percent of black and 1.5 percent of Hispanic people) (Gust, Darling, Kennedy, and Schwartz 2008, 721; Omer et al. 2009). This often is due to unproven vaccine safety concerns. For other populations, previous experience of discrimination and medical deception also contribute (see Chapter 2).

Understandings about some of the ingredients used to manufacture immunization compounds (e.g., blood serum from cattle or horses) likewise can stand in the way of acceptance due to incompatibility with cultural beliefs about what should or should not enter the body. Beliefs about penetration of body boundaries (e.g., the skin) likewise may lead some to shun immunization. These issues must be respectfully anticipated by anyone involved in an immunization campaign.

Sometimes, merely the provision of alternate routes of inoculation (e.g., oral ingestion) or of preparations without any offending ingredients, or patiently explaining that what the refusee thinks is in the vaccine actually is not, is enough to change refusal to agreement.

NUTRITIONAL CONCERNS

In addition to exposure to infectious diseases, babies are vulnerable to other hazards that cultural practices can exacerbate or mitigate. For example, infants are vulnerable to infections and malnutrition that can be prevented by breast milk, which provides antibodies and proper nourishment. When mothers no longer nurse their young due to the development and use of infant formulas, infants can lose some degree of this naturally conferred immunity.

Another reason to breastfeed, especially in poor populations, is that diarrheal diseases can be better avoided if no formula is given. Formula often is mixed with unclean water and given in unsterilized bottles or cups. Contaminated water and utensils can trouble the gut, and malnutrition results when food is not kept in the digestive tract long enough to be absorbed. Further, formula often is diluted by poor mothers who need to stretch it, meaning that nutrients taken in would not, even if absorbed, be enough to provide a good nutritive start for the infant (Moore et al. 1980, 124). Research using a large nationally representative sample concluded that breastfeeding could save about 720 infants each year from dying (Chen and Rogan 2004, e435).

THE TRIALS OF CHILDHOOD

SPECIAL HEALTH CARE NEEDS

Those children who make it through infancy still can have health challenges to face. Today, over 10 million (13.9 percent) U.S. children have a significant ongoing health care need. One in five households are affected. Allergies, asthma, attention deficit hyperactivity disorder or ADHD, autism, cerebral palsy, cystic fibrosis, diabetes, Down syndrome, emotional problems, headaches, mental retardation, and muscular dystrophy are among the most common conditions reported. Top functional difficulties include respiratory problems; learning and behavior problems; anxiety or depression; problems speaking, communicating, or being understood; chronic pain; gross and fine motor challenges; and problems swallowing, digesting food, or with metabolism (Data Resource Center for Child and Adolescent Health 2009).

Benefits notwithstanding, in addition to the various kinds of costs such conditions have for children are the costs entailed for families, many of which are overwhelmed by the challenges faced in simply learning to navigate the health care system to optimize care for their children, let alone by the financial burdens they bear. On top of this, the effort of advocating for their children can take a heavy toll. Parents can find themselves in a complicated bind in which love of and hope for their children compete with negative cultural views of the children's conditions—views shaped by U.S. ideals regarding physical and mental perfection, individual accomplishment, social adulthood, and so forth. These negative views (internalized to a greater or lesser extent by different parents) both fuel biomedicine's curative stance, and compete with more positive disability rights movement and generic Judeo-Christian views about the value of every individual.

One strategy parents of children with Down syndrome who participated in an interview study reported using to deal with this issue involved framing their experiences as transformational opportunities to become better people through devoted parenting. They also deployed religious imagery, for example, calling a child with Down syndrome "a gift from God." Disability rights rhetoric promoting the value of physical diversity also is used in this way. The practice of labeling disabled children as *exceptional* and *special* draws strength here (Sobo 2010).

Injury and Abuse

Despite the existence of chronic conditions, childhood is generally a time of learning and anticipatory socialization for the life ahead. It is also the stage at which good health habits can be developed, such as adequate practices of diet, exercise, dental care, and body awareness. Now that major infectious diseases are generally under control, the major cause of death among children is injuries—primarily unintentional injuries occurring from motor vehicle crashes (U.S. Department of Health and Human Services 1992, 12). Preventive care needs to go beyond immunizations, and recognition and treatment of early problems. It needs to include raising awareness of possible hazards, such as poisoning and drowning, and encouraging proper use of automobile seat belts or restraining devices.

Childhood illness and injury are strongly associated with poverty and low educational levels. These can make proper nutrition, exercise, and preventive health care impossible. Since resulting health problems may produce long-term conditions such as mental retardation, learning disorders, behavioral problems, and sensory impairments, "an accurate profile of the health of US children ... must also consider emotional, psychological, and learning problems, the social and environmental risks to which they are related, and the total costs to the Nation" (U.S. Department of Health and Human Services 1992, 12).

A tremendous problem for children across cultures is intentional injury and abuse. Abuse includes neglect, withholding or delaying medical treatment, and outright violent attack. While violence affects us at all levels of the life course, abuse of children is particularly deplorable because of the power disparity in the adult-child relationship. The effects of child abuse last a lifetime and affect victims' abilities to function as healthy adults (see Widom 1989).

Nearly 800,000 children are abused or neglected per year, according to official case statistics—which do not include countless unreported or officially unresolved cases. Children aged one year or less have the highest rates (about 30/1000), and girls account for slightly more victims than boys. Neglect is most common, followed by physical, then sexual, then psychological maltreatment (U.S. Department of Health and Human Services 2009, xii–xiii). Much abuse is found in poor families; however, "any correlation between abuse and poverty is biased by the fact that the behavior of the poor is more likely to be reported in official records than that of members of other classes, who are better equipped to conceal their activities" (Kornblum and Julian 1995, 211).

Although domestic abuse seems to be most common in industrialized nations, it also exists in other societies, including small-scale ones (Korbin 1987; Soroka and Bryjak 1995, 315–17). Developing nations, due to greater concerns over disease and malnutrition, are only beginning to see maltreatment of children as an issue to be addressed (Korbin 1987).

Treatment of children should always be understood within a cultural context, as should the definition of "harm." However, argues Korbin (1987), "any practice, whether collective or individual, that compromises children's development and survival must be critically considered. Practices that inflict potential physical or psychic pain and harm on all children, or all children in particular categories, must be subjected to empirical tests of harm and not judged on an implicit or explicit ethnocentric basis" (29). Harming children (like harming anyone) must not be accepted as a culturally relative practice justified by tradition.

Korbin states that "cultural competence challenges ethnocentric beliefs about what is good for children or what is abusive and neglectful. It also furthers knowledge of the circumstances under which child abuse and neglect are most likely to occur and, in turn, most likely to be prevented" (1987, 35).

Several factors placing children at risk for abuse are identified across cultures: deformities or handicaps and multiple or difficult births, which may be interpreted as malevolent or inauspicious; culturally defined illegitimacy; gender preferences; rapid socioeconomic and sociocultural change; urbanization; stress; unemployment; and poverty. The fact that immigrant children may become knowledgeable and acculturate to a new environment more rapidly than parents and become less obedient and compliant also may come into play (Korbin 1987).

The American Medical Association (AMA) provides medical guidelines for identifying and handling domestic abuse. Health care providers must comply with laws where abuse is suspected, but they can also inform themselves regarding supportive networks and agencies such as churches, shelters, and other advocates for battered women and children, and provide appropriate referrals. Additional resources and referrals may be necessary since children are themselves becoming more involved as protagonists in violent behavior, creating further problems for providing care.

Since the traditional biomedical system addresses cure rather than prevention, the focus is on treating conditions after they occur. The preventability of many childhood medical problems vividly illustrates the inadequacy of this type of approach. Physicians, however, are beginning to participate as advocates of preventive programs. The AMA and other medical organizations have thrown their weight behind a number of public health campaigns and related legislation. Their goals have included the prevention of cigarette smoking in children, the elimination of dangerous exposure to secondhand smoke, and the promotion of seat belt use in automobiles, trigger locks on guns, and helmets on bike, scooter, and skateboard riders.

ADOLESCENCE

Violence is not confined to children; adolescents also are abused, and they abuse others. In our society, this is tied in part to the cultural view of adolescence as a time for risk taking and dramatics. However, as Margaret Mead (1963 [1928]) showed so many years ago, adolescence need not be a time of great "sturm und drang"—it certainly was not stormy for the Samoan adolescents involved in her research. For them, "adolescence represented no period of crisis or stress" (95), partly because of the "general casualness" (117) of Samoan culture and partly because of a cultural value on conflict avoidance.

Despite cultural differences, adolescence "is everywhere associated with pubertal events such as menstruation, the appearance of secondary sexual features ... or general changes in body conformation," write Schlegel and Barry (1991, 198–99), whose major cross-cultural study of adolescence was the first of its kind. After systematically investigating compiled data from 186 societies, the researchers concluded that adolescence is indeed a universal life stage, albeit one that varies according to a group's economic, familial, and social structural organization.

Adolescence also varies by gender: Generally it lasts longer for boys than for girls, who may enter the status of adult earlier than boys do, through pregnancy or marriage (Schlegel and Barry 1991, 12). Girls also experience their growth spurt (e.g., in height) and reproductive maturation closer together in time than do boys (Moore et al. 1980, 138). And they have the very demarcated experience of menarche, the first menstrual flow, while for boys physical puberty is a more nebulous event. In Europe and the United States, menarche now occurs about 2 years earlier than it did 100 years ago. Worldwide, it occurs earlier in urban areas and among the wealthy. These trends seem to be linked to better nutrition and increased body fat (139–40). Emotional maturity, however, may be less developed.

YOUTHFUL RISK TAKING

Adolescence is also a time of exploration, and this sometimes involves risk taking. This can be noted with initiation of sexual activity. By ninth grade, 34.3 percent of U.S. students have reported ever having had sexual intercourse; by tenth, 42.8 percent; by eleventh 51.4 percent; and by twelfth, 63.1 percent (CDC 2006, 19). Nationwide, 33.9 percent of students reported having had sexual intercourse with one or more people in the past three months prior to being surveyed (20). Among these, 23.3 percent had drunk alcohol or used drugs before having sex; 62.8 percent reported having used a condom (21).

Without barrier protection, youths are vulnerable to a range of sexually transmitted conditions, including pregnancy and HIV infection. Factual education alone is not the answer. There seems to be little relation between knowledge of sexual risks and decreased risky behavior (Hingson and Strunin 1992, 24). This is in part because adolescents in America are socialized to take sexual risks. There are many cultural reasons for doing so, one being that such behavior confers status and self-esteem (see Sobo 1995). It may also not be perceived as "risky."

Further, what is risky in one situation might not be as risky in another. For example, while pregnant teens in middle-class neighborhoods might have little practical experience in child care and might have many opportunities for further education, an inner-city teen will likely have spent a great deal of time caring for others' babies and will probably not even have the same educational chances that middle-class girls who bear children will consequently lose.

Youthful risk taking in the United States goes beyond sex to include substance use—the use of drugs, tobacco, or alcohol—often in combination with driving, which is, for many youths, a symbol of maturity and so an eagerly approached activity. When we pair this with the finding that 30 percent of youth reported having ridden with an alcohol-drinking driver in the month prior to being asked, the trend toward texting even while driving, and the fact that 18 percent never or rarely use seat belts (CDC 2009b, 33), it is no surprise that automobile accidents are a major cause of death and disability among adolescents.

Intervention must take place early and it should go beyond simple factual health messages to address broader cultural issues that surround risky activities. For example, teens could be reminded that smoking causes bad breath, which others find offensive. The opinions of others, however, could also promote the habit: Some teens smoke to stay thin. Because of cultural values, the fear of fat may override any fears about personal offense or even possible lung cancer (Hechinger 1992, 11). Education for a healthy diet as well as to build self-esteem may do the most good here.

Care after the fact involves recognition, sensitivity, building trust, and referral skills in the health care provider. Confidentiality also must be assured; adolescents' fear of breaches in confidentiality may keep them from telling practitioners about their substance use or other sensitive matters. In a Massachusetts study, 25 percent of high school students reported that they would forgo health care in some situations if they thought that their parents might find out (Cheng, Savageua, Sattler, and DeWitt 1993, 1404).

SUICIDE

Another major cause of death among youths—12 percent, in fact (CDC/NCDPHP 2009)—is suicide. Suicide generally has complex roots. It can, for instance, stem from a crisis related to an adolescent's worries about being homo- or bisexual (where such identities are stigmatized). Indeed, in the United States, gay and lesbian youth are two to three times more likely to attempt suicide than heterosexual youth, and such suicide attempts are "more serious and more lethal than those of their heterosexual peers" (Messina 1992, 1; see also Silenzio et al. 2007). Among heterosexual youth, drug use and depression are key predictors (Silenzio et al. 2007). Health care providers may have an impact on the suicide problem simply through increased awareness. In the case of nonheterosexual youth, showing sensitivity and concern, rather than denial or condemnation is key.

ADULTHOOD

RESPONSIBILITY FOR SELF AND OTHERS

Independent adults have more opportunity than infants, children, adolescents, or older people to take responsibility for their health. Many of the leading causes of death in adults are preventable, often through lifestyle changes. The decline in rates of coronary heart disease and stroke deaths, both of which have dropped by about half since 1970, is in a large part due to a decrease in cigarette smoking and an increased attention to diet and to controlling high blood pressure. Over the same time period, adult automobile accident death rates declined by about one-third. This was due to more seat belt use, less alcohol use, and lowered speed limits. Social and behavioral changes—and cultural changes that supported them—thus affected adults' health status (Public Health Service 1992, 19). Also during adulthood, poor or toxic working conditions, high stress levels, alcohol and tobacco use, depression and despair all may take their toll, especially on poor (including homeless) adults who, due to their position in the social structure, have little agency or control over their lives. Women also may, in some societies, be added to this group due to gender constructions by which they find themselves restricted, powerless, and/or isolated.

Still, adults generally have more autonomy than youths, and more authority enabling them to influence, for instance via voting, health policies, and laws that can affect specific populations or society in general. Adults in power can make or repeal laws dealing with pollution, risky behavior, or safe food supplies and consumer goods. However, all adults face various health problems particular to their life stage, as well as those related to behaviors and lifestyles undertaken in their earlier years.

MENOPAUSE: BIOLOGY AND CULTURE

Gender differences affecting the meaning of adulthood can be quite profound. In some societies, women who are social adults still have only the rights of children, and can make few decisions for themselves.

In some cultures, this changes after women undergo menopause (e.g., among the Hua; see Meigs 1983), the logic being that now that they do not menstruate and cannot bear children they are more like men and therefore should have similar rights. Of course, in other contexts, postmenopausal women may be seen not so much "as good as" men, but rather as "lesser" women (see Chapter 2).

Because of cultural norms for female bodies, postmenopausal women in the United States may interpret changes, such as facial hair growth or a lowering of vocal pitch, as masculinization. Age-linked infertility may be distressing for women in certain cultural contexts, where women's value hinges on their childbearing function. But it also can come as a relief.

Menopause itself is very nebulous process. The label of "menopause" however, constructs what is partly a social transition as a purely biological transition. Biomedical specialists define menopause technically as the occurrence of the last menstrual period, making it an "event in time" (Kaufert 1986, 333). However, women cross-culturally experience it as a process that takes place over time, and they use a "self-anchoring definition" (333) of menopause, seeing themselves as menopausal when there has been a change in their bodily patterns, for example, in the menstrual cycle.

The biomedical definition of menopause is used in a scientific context, because a woman's last menstrual period provides a relatively easy index across populations. Signs and symptoms are more ambiguous, however, and because a woman's own definitions may be equally valid, the physician's role should not be to define, but to distinguish between the pathological and the nonpathological in the patient (Kaufert 1986, 76).

The physician also needs to bear in mind that there are many reasons besides menopause that might account for menstrual changes (which are but one sign of menopause). Indeed, as Patricia Kaufert notes, "a model based on the well-nourished women of the white middle class is clearly inappropriate to societies where women are frequently malnourished or constantly overburdened by pregnancy or physical or psychological stress. Under these conditions menstruation becomes sparse and irregular well before the expected age of menopause" (1986, 335).

Although the average age of 50 is remarkably universal for onset of menopause, a survey of 30 societies conducted before the recent and potentially confounding surge of globalization revealed that only in two societies besides the United States was the event seen as a major physical and emotional loss (Bart 1969). The accompanying symptoms of distress found in the United States were not even noted in other societies such as in India (Flint 1975).

Medically, not only women but also men undergo "menopause." For men, who do not have such a visible sign of fecundity as the menstrual period, menopause is "a far more dubious entity" (Katchadourian 1978, 47). As with women, hormone balances gradually change. Testicular function gradually declines and men experience an attendant loss in potency and fertility. In the United States, these changes are not culturally recognized; they challenge sociocultural concepts of both masculinity and femininity. There is no medical specialty for male sexual problems, which are instead included under the specialty of urology.

THE AGING POPULATION

GROWING OLD CULTURALLY

Aging is unpopular in the United States. Although the number of older citizens is increasing rapidly, the cultural emphasis is still on the youthful image. Products are constantly emerging in the marketplace to erase or minimize wrinkles, color or replace hair, provide boundless energy, improve memory, and boost sexual prowess and performance. Some of these products and procedures, such as plastic surgery, face lifts, varicose vein removal, tummy tucks, and liposuction, are obtained within or from the medical institution. The market for such treatments and services is expanding as the aging population continues to grow.

The fact that more and more people are living to their 70s and 80s, plus the unprecedented rise in birth rates after World War II (the baby boom cohort) means that we will see a large bulge in the retirement population somewhere between 2015 and 2030 (Atchley 1994, 44–45). The resulting changes in proportions in age categories will have profound consequences for the restructuring of health care.

Those age 85 and up (the old-old) are the fastest-growing segment of the population, estimated to increase from 2.3 percent in 2010, to 5.2 percent by 2050 (Thorson, 2000, 12–14). There will be more elderly women, because (unless the ratios change) women outlive men by about seven to eight years. The old-old (mostly women) will also be more likely than others to live in nursing homes and to have substantial disabilities and extremely limited financial resources. Even though at present most older people do receive care and assistance from spouses and families, that arrangement may change. More people do not marry or have children; families have grown smaller; their human as well as financial resources have shrunk (see Chapter 2).

Although aging is not a disease any more than is childhood, adolescence, or adulthood, the last years of our lives carry a higher risk of chronic ailments, some of which may have taken root at an earlier time in the life course. A lifetime of poverty and distress, including a work history of part-time, low-paying, physically demanding or hazardous jobs, with few benefits and perhaps many periods without wages will lead to more health problems and fewer resources at old age. Thus being old and poor, or old and poor and female, or old and poor and female and minority, compounds the problems of aging.

CULTURAL MEANINGS OF AGE: THE MAINSTREAM

In many societies, wisdom and authority are attributed to the elderly who, through life experience, have gained social standing and achieved the right to respect. They are also seen as a major resource in teaching others how to understand the world and to survive.

Cultural views of aging in the United States are tied to historical and social-structural factors as well as related ideals and values. The negative connotations of aging came with modernization. Before the American Revolution, older, free, white males from the appropriate social class owned property, directed the family, and therefore had much control within the community and held advantages in trade, politics, and religion. There were fewer elderly; age was considered granted by God's favor and therefore venerated.

With modernization and industrialization, however, there is a concomitant loss of roles for the elderly. The wisdom of age becomes obsolete; civil authority is dispersed to younger citizens; there is an expansion of wealth and trade. Land ownership becomes less important with growth of industry and urbanization (Cowgill 1972).

Atchley (1994), however, proposes that it is social ideology more than objective reality that has influenced our perceptions of aging. The ideals of equality attacked the moral basis for a hierarchical, age-graded society even before that equality was declared. Further, as modernization increased its pace, older people were culturally cast as obsolete.

In any case, with modernization, improved standards of living and medical care extended life expectancy. More people began to live longer. By the 1930s, the Social Security program was created to provide a motivation for retirement through the provision of benefits funded by taxes paid by the worker, freeing up jobs for younger citizens as well as offering a cushion for retirees. Ironically, Social Security contributed to a vision of the aging as less capable and unable to manage by—or speak for—themselves.

This vision has influenced how aging people are treated in nursing homes as well as in general. Athena McLean has shown how facility residents' refusal to tolerate demeaning or dehumanizing treatment, often demonstrated by withdrawal or noncooperative and sometimes disruptive behavior, can be cast by nursing home staff and providers as medically rooted rather than socioculturally generated. It therefore is treated by pharmaceutical means; in other words, those who speak or act up are sedated (2007).

In many ways, the medical institution contributed to the developing cultural view that denies elders a voice. This view casts aging as a time of increasing dependency and decrepitude, with expectations of aches and pains, memory loss, and other concomitant conditions. Biological research on the aging process characterized it as decline and degeneration.

Paradoxically, modernization also produced better general living conditions and longer life expectancy. The older population increasingly has refused to accept aging as obsolescence. In response to the needs and demands of a growing elderly population, new discoveries and research on aging have contributed to a healthier, more active, and hence even larger population of citizens at the far end of life.

AGING OUTSIDE OF THE MAINSTREAM

From a multicultural perspective, the status and treatment of the elderly is more complex. Native Americans are a case in point. It is impossible to generalize about the Native American, because tribes vary extensively in relation to language and customs, location, history, and so forth; there is also variation within tribes. However, most values related to aging and the elderly among Native Americans are connected with having useful roles and being able to fulfill them. In the past, older Native Americans' roles included caring for grandchildren and passing knowledge down to the young. Some were midwives or healers and religious specialists; many were leaders. Power and prestige derived from patterns of land ownership and economic production that favored the old (Schweitzer 1983).

Today, the problems of older Native Americans parallel those of other minority or impoverished elderly. Besides poverty, itself a powerful predictor of poor outcomes, the loss of roles, and of respect for elder knowledge, as the young move into the larger society and traditions are lost, has created a type of **anomie**, or loss of meaning, and the result for many has been isolation, alcoholism, disease, and despair (Kunitz 1983).

BIOMEDICINE, CHANGE, AND THE ELDERLY

The modern U.S. health care system was built on the model of military medicine for acute care (see Chapter 5). It came of age at a time when infectious disease was losing its grip as a major killer. U.S. health care standards reflect the historical assumption that care will be for specific, discrete, acute, curable conditions. Today, however, chronic care accounts for the bulk of U.S. care utilization and spending. The change from acute infectious disease to chronic degenerative diseases as a major cause of death in this century has had huge implications for health care.

Chronic care, particularly for the elderly, requires more cooperation and understanding between doctor and patient, as well as family, when present. As people age, there is a greater need to monitor intake of medications, capacities for self-care, and understanding of and agreement with treatment regimens. For many years, cultural attitudes about the elderly as well as about growing old were reflected in biomedicine, which viewed the needs and changes in capacities of the aging mind and body as simply inevitable and generally not matters for medical intervention. As the population ages, the role of medicine will be tied to other institutions in determining quality, as much as quantity of life for the aging.

DEATH: THE FINAL STAGE OF MORTAL LIFE

Dying is not optional. Cultural factors, however, influence the types and rates of illness, both physical and mental, as well as causes of death in all cultural groups. Further, all cultures devise different ways to deal with death—complete with explanations, grieving procedures, celebrations, and rituals.

In Western culture, death has become institutionalized and hidden; the focus has shifted away from the dead to others' response to the demise of loved ones. Survivors attempt to hide emotions, the body is whisked off to the mortician's offices immediately, the coffin becomes a "casket," the body is embalmed to give the appearance of being life-like or natural, and mourning is carefully orchestrated to the visitation and funeral (Corr, Nabe, and Corr 1997, 71–72). The standardization of certain aspects of the modern rituals of death, such as disposal of the body, is now based upon public health concerns and therefore subject to law.

In the United States, the vast majority of deaths take place in the hospital, often alone, rather than in a domestic space surrounded by family and friends. Survivors rarely see the bodies of the dead except fleetingly. They generally do not touch them. These cultural practices send messages about core American values, such as the focus on sanitation, emotional control, and individuality (cf. Turner 1995).

Other conceptualizations, however, do exist. Like birth and other significant passages in the life course, dying and death are accompanied with a myriad of social and cultural meanings and rituals. Attending to traditions can be comforting and an essential part of the grieving process. It is important, therefore, for health care workers confronted with death to encourage the dying and their survivors to attend to practices that are important to them.

DEATH IN A SUBCULTURE

Although personal variations may be considerable, representing a large number of intervening variables, grieving styles can differ from group to group and cultural tendencies are best treated with understanding and sensitivity. For example, Galanti (2008, 175–76) describes the case of a young Vietnamese man who was found clinically dead after an accident. He was placed on a ventilator until the family could be notified. When the family arrived, they informed the physician that they wished to keep the man on life support until the "right time" for his death. They had consulted an astrologer who advised waiting. Within a week, they announced that he could die and the ventilator was discontinued.

Astrology is taken very seriously by many Asians, as well as some other groups. Dying at the "right time," notes Galanti, signifies good fortune for the descendants of the deceased. Otherwise, the children will suffer negative fates. In this case, the family had a chance to avert this outcome.

The physician and medical staff in this case were stunned by the incident and sought information through books on astrology and through Vietnamese coworkers. They realized that cultural beliefs and values are a very real part of people's lives. Although it is not always possible to honor those beliefs and values, concessions can often be made and the remedy may be as simple as a screen for privacy or allowing for cultural rituals.

DEATH AND BIOMEDICINE

There is some speculation that a fear of or inability to deal with death leads some individuals into the field of biomedicine. The doctor becomes St. George (or Georgia), battling the enemy death, the dragon. When death occurs, however, it is often seen as failure on the part of the doctor.

Death has become medicalized and is managed and controlled by physicians, at least up to the point when a patient is defined as "dying" (Muller and Koenig 1988, 371). That particular point seems to be key in determining the role and participation of physicians in the care of seriously ill (and perhaps dying) patients. Muller and Koenig (1988) found that medical interns tended not to define a patient as dying, as long as there was something—*anything*—to do (i.e., to treat), or the physician viewed (or constructed) the patient as "having a chance." Once the patient has been defined as "dying," doctors may feel they have nothing more to do. The patient is labeled a "futile case"; the doctors then tend to disappear, leaving the dying to nurses and family.

But the point at which a patient is defined as dying may not be the same point at which patient or family recognize death as imminent.

Patients (or their proxies) may decide to reject further treatment and ask to be allowed to die at home among friends and family or in a hospice setting. The hospice philosophy includes numerous points, but primary among these are holistic care to the patient and family as a unit, and helping the patient live until death occurs—not extending the dying process while the patient lives. Care includes ongoing teamwork that is directed to the patient and family's various needs, including pain control with adequate doses of pain medication, withdrawal of active treatment, home care where possible, the provision of a human and loving environment that affirms life and allows death, and continuing support of bereaved family after the death (Corr, Nabe, and Corr 1997, 199–200). This philosophy is notably in conflict with the biomedical ideal of never giving up the fight for life, and seeing death as failure.

Not only is the point at which a person can be called "dying" rather nebulous; so too is the point of death itself. For most of time and across most cultures, death was signified by cessation of breathing and heartbeat. However, the notion of "brain death" was introduced in the 1960s when life support technologies had been developed and interest in and the possibility of organ transplantation or "transfer" (Sharp 2006) was on the rise. In addition to medical breakthroughs, organ transfer was increasingly possible due to other breakthroughs; for instance, with more people driving, and cars able to go faster, more car crashes happened and these produced more sudden deaths among people whose organs were otherwise quite healthy and vital.

The invention of the diagnosis of whole-brain death helped to support the organ transfer process (Lock 2002). The diagnosis means that all brain activity has permanently ceased. However, the rest of a brain-dead person's body parts must be kept alive for a time after whole-brain death has been confirmed so that the organs remain useable for transplant purposes. To this end, the heart of an individual who is technically dead can be kept pumping and blood oxygenated with mechanical means.

North American rationalism supports the equation made between the person and the mind and, by extension, the brain. However, to others, such as the Japanese, the idea is nonsensical at best. In Japan, the vital essence of the person is not equated solely with the mind-brain; instead, the person infuses the body as a whole, residing in the anatomically nonspecific *kokoro* (Lock 2002).

Partly for this reason, despite their high-tech reputation, the Japanese have been very hesitant to embrace organ transplantation. As Lock argues, it simply does not have a good cultural fit (2002).

Moreover, each person is connected in important ways to other persons in his or her social network. Ancestors (the dead) remain an important part of this network, so to cut up their bodies would be disrespectful and socially disruptive. Concurrently, although North American medical practice conforms to a theory of individual autonomy—by which individuals have full rights to determine their disposition after death—Japanese practice does not: The family has that right and must be consulted. Indeed, to some degree, the family even has the right to determine when a family member is dead; doctors often wait until they have had time to come to terms with a death before proclaiming it, and thus legally creating it (Lock 2002).

IN THE END

As the technological possibilities change and multiply, more choices will have to be made. Social values, including the values of independent choice, family involvement, the value placed on "life," how life is to be defined, the weighing of economic priorities as well as supply versus demand, the consequences of medical intervention or no medical intervention—all must be considered in health care decision making by patients, families, and providers.

When biomedicine fails to meet our human and cultural needs, we may look elsewhere for care and support. In the following chapter, we examine other available systems that offer alternative or complementary modalities that, for various reasons, people may feel better suit their needs and expectations.

FOR DISCUSSION

1. How does the cultural construction of the life course affect the possibilities of health and illness in a population? How can awareness of life course issues be used in providing health care?

2. What should be the role of the health care practitioner, including physician, in dealing with personal and structural causal factors in illness at each level of the life course? Why should the practitioner be concerned with nonbiomedical factors?

3. Generally speaking, what changes have taken place in the American life course that relate to health and illness? What changes will most probably take place in the near future? How might they affect the delivery of health care?

CHAPTER 4

Therapeutic Modalities: A Cross-Cultural Perspective

GOAL: Describe the diversity of ways in which humans view the body and its workings, conceptualize illness, and provide health care within differentiated and sometimes overlapping systems.

GOAL: Demonstrate that there are various approaches to healing and various categories of healers; describe some of the key differences and similarities in both approaches and categories.

GOAL: Explain and exemplify how various approaches to healing and categories of healers may be complementary.

It is easy to make intellectual errors when dealing with medical systems. We forget that our own perspectives may prevent us from understanding the meaning and utility of practices that have been developed within another culture. That failure to account for our own needs and biases also can lead to the overenthusiastic acceptance of ideas whose genesis and application we really do not understand.

(Ergil 1996, 185)

When Jennifer began feeling lethargic and her occasional migraine headaches became more frequent, she thought perhaps it was just the stress of work. However, when her problems began to affect her work, a close friend recommended that she see a homeopath, Dr. Senseman, who had successfully treated him. Jennifer had never heard of homeopathy, but decided to give it a try. Dr. Senseman took a comprehensive history, allowing Jennifer to talk for over an hour, and then prescribed a remedy delivered in tiny white sugar pills. Within a week, Jennifer was feeling much better, and the headaches had not returned.

Jennifer's case reminds us that there are a multitude of ways we may perceive or respond to pain or illness. What is available to us and what we choose to do and why are inextricably context-bound. The social structure allows or provides one or numerous alternatives, and our own socialization, enculturation, and past experience provide our motivation for action. This chapter compares and contrasts the various ways that cultures influence us in perceiving illness and meeting health needs.

HEALTH CARE CATEGORIES

Several scholars have created typologies that attempt to describe the range and use of various therapeutic systems or **modalities** and to highlight related cultural issues. Despite best intentions, most typologies are founded on ethnocentric assumptions, such as the primacy or superiority of one system over another. This is not in all cases a fatal flaw. We all have biases. The trick is to try to understand our biases and to anticipate how they may be reflected in thoughts and actions. As long as the assumptions in the frameworks we use to understand other people's choices are acknowledged, and the reasons for our adhering to them made clear, they may still facilitate our thinking about health issues.

Another problem with health typologies is that they are descriptive but generally not explanatory. People using them may become so concerned with categorizing or naming things in accordance with the scheme at hand that they lose sight of the goal of understanding the various classified elements. And schemes applied cross-culturally can be problematic because they ask us to evaluate cultural traits or items in a way that divorces them from their cultural context (cf. Augé and Herzlich 1995).

Further, classification schemes by definition fragment reality, carving it up into small components. This can camouflage the fact that the elements together might form a system, the whole of which is greater than the sum of its single parts. It also can, when some components are downplayed, present a picture that is partial at best: For instance, most schemes do not take into account the backstage of health care. They focus on healers while actually the majority of health care workers occupy behind-the-scenes nonclinical roles (e.g., administration, facilities support, food services). Finally, many health events or care approaches straddle the lines

Table 4.1
Medical modalities: Some key typologies

Kleinman (1978)
Professional (e.g., biomedicine, Ayurveda)
Folk (e.g., faith healing, shamanism)
Popular (e.g., mother's care)

O'Connor (1995)
Conventional (dominative systems; e.g., biomedicine in the United States,
    acupuncture in China)
Vernacular (e.g., mother's care, faith healing)

Wardwell (1972)
Biomedical (e.g., licensed MDs; nurses)
Adjunct (e.g., medical technicians)
Limited (e.g., dentists)
Marginal (e.g., chiropractors)
Quasi-medical (e.g., faith healers; quacks)

Young (1983)
Accumulating (e.g., biomedicine, Ayurveda)
Diffusing (e.g., shamanism)

---

set forth in the classification schemes. In many cases, it is helpful to think of categories as having a continuum running between them. Several major categorization schemes are represented in Table 4.1.

THE THREE MEDICAL SECTORS

One common typology is Arthur Kleinman's tripartite scheme of popular, folk, and professional medicine (1986a [1978]). In this scheme, which is meant to subsume not only biomedical but other approaches to healing, there are three sectors of health care, and the key variables are who provides care, and in what context. **Popular**-sector treatment is based on shared cultural understandings and is provided by nonspecialists, like one's self, one's mother, one's friends, or other kin and relations. **Folk**-sector healers are specialists whose practice is based on traditional methods and philosophies. Legally sanctioned official systems (e.g., biomedical) make up the **professional** sector.

This typology has been immensely helpful for thinking about medical care. It is an advance on simple "public-private" dichotomizing, in which private or household care is generally bounded as completely separate and is discounted. It allows for the interpenetration of these two arenas, and values events that take place in the home. However, the division of labor by gender is not considered, which downplays the large contribution of women. The terms chosen also are problematic, at least taken at face value.

Kleinman's model specifically allows that some nonbiomedical practices, such as Ayurvedic medicine in India (soon described) and chiropractic, should be classed as professional-sector offerings due to their routinized, formalized, professionalized nature. However, this is easily forgotten by those who would view those therapeutic modalities as folk practices.

O'Connor (1995), who has noted that there is some stigma carried in the term "folk," with its insinuation of undereducation, superstition, and mistaken understandings, provides a corrective in a model that has only two parts: conventional medicine and vernacular medicine. **Vernacular** medicine subsumes Kleinman's (1986a [1978]) folk and popular sectors; **conventional** medicine consists only of the official, authorized, authoritative, dominative health care industry or system—whatever that may be in a given cultural context. The contrast is simple but important, because it explicitly highlights the dominative position held by conventional medicine (seen in the fact that we often just call it "medicine"). The power dynamics and medical status hierarchy that O'Connor's model reflects are, to at least some extent, universal (all systems have conventional medicine of some kind).

Of course, in some societies, no healing practices are professionalized and all are quite informal. As Gilbert Lewis explains, "There may be no separation of a department of knowledge and practice specifically orientated towards human sickness. Illness may be treated by religious or other specialists as one of their many duties; the explanations to account for it may stem from theories or premises that have much wider relevance than to sickness alone" (1986, 135). Further, the apparent orderliness of some nonbiomedical traditions may in fact be an artifact of modernization, which demands an emphasis on rational systems.

And so, while Kleinman's tripartite scheme remains relevant to the current organization of health care in the United States, the notions of a distinct health system that is internally systematic and of professionalization are somewhat culture-bound. This limits the universal applicability of the scheme, as does the fact that the scheme has only three parts. There are many different types of healers in our folk and professional sectors, and a more elaborate scheme may be necessary if we are to fully understand the internal workings of these systems.

WARDWELL'S TYPOLOGY: RELATIONS WITH BIOMEDICINE

A slightly more complex but biomedically centered scheme was devised by Wardwell (1972). This typology reflects Wardwell's position as a sociologist, for medical sociology had much firmer links within biomedicine when it took root than did medical anthropology. In fact, Wardwell's scheme dealt mostly with groups struggling for conventional power and status. Thus, the scheme included limited practitioners, such as pharmacists, podiatrists, dentists, optometrists, and clinical psychologists. Limited practitioners were seen as independent of, but accepted by, the medical profession, and each type treated particular areas of the human body.

Marginal practitioners generally treated a full range of disorders, but used therapies unacceptable to medical professionals. These practitioners included chiropractors, homeopaths, naturopaths, reflexologists, acupuncturists, and formerly osteopaths, who have since moved into the biomedical sector. Acupuncturists and chiropractors have also moved along the scale, becoming licensed and included in some insurance plans. The key to the so-called marginality of these practitioners resides mostly in the fact that they tend to reject the biomedical approaches and support monocausal theories of illness (e.g., chiropractors hold that the major cause of illness is misalignment of the spine). They also generally shun the use of drugs as poisons and often have a tradition of hostility toward biomedical practitioners.

Unconventional groups, such as "quacks" (fraudulent medical practitioners), faith healers, magical healers, and the like were classed as "quasi-practitioners." The therapies of quasi-practitioners were seen as pseudoscientific, nonmedical, and often incidental to another, possibly religious, function. There are long traditions behind these healers, whose success is seen as mainly psychotherapeutic. Any psychotherapeutic benefits, however, have generally not been recognized by the biomedical profession, which tends to see most of these systems as exploitative. Further, empirically validated traditional systems outside of biomedicine are not included in Wardwell's scheme.

Wardwell's typology continues to be of use in tracking social change's effects on health care through its focus on the relationships between therapeutic modalities. We would, however, suggest revising the classification scheme to include biomedicine as but one sector of the typology, including physicians, nurses, psychiatrists, physician's assistants, nurse practitioners, emergency medical technicians, and so on. We also would add an "adjunct" classification to include post-1970s service providers such as radiologists, X-ray technicians, physical therapists, respiratory therapists, and others whose functions are assistant to biomedicine.

With the use of a more balanced and expanded typology, it should be possible to discern other patterns, such as growth or decline, and shortcomings and advantages of changing modalities. The typology can also be useful in tracking cross-referential complementary interactions (e.g., physicians who refer to chiropractors, chiropractors and physicians who practice homeopathy or acupuncture, faith healers and shamans who work with physicians, etc.) Examining this interaction can help us to identify the various dimensions of human need, complementarity, and the various outcomes when therapies are combined.

ACCUMULATING AND DIFFUSING MEDICINES

Alan Young (1983) recognized that biomedicine was not a universal yardstick for measuring all other systems. He instead divided all medical systems according to whether they entailed accumulated, formalized teachings or, rather, encouraged the fragmentation and diffusion of medical knowledge.

Accumulating and diffusing systems can be seen as on a continuum. **Accumulating** systems involve the collection of knowledge, generally in written form, conferences at which knowledge is shared, professional associations, and institutions for formal training. Biomedicine is an extreme version of an accumulating system. Chinese medicine, Ayurveda, Unani, and Galenic systems of medicine (all to be described) are also accumulating systems. **Diffusing** systems, on the other hand, do not have forums for communication between practitioners. Knowledge often is guarded as secret and rarely shared. Some shamans and magical healers working on their own are participants in diffusing systems (Young 1983, 1206). While this typology is limited by its simplicity, it demonstrates how looking at medicine from a different angle can open up new options for cross-cultural comparisons.

ANATOMY AND PHYSIOLOGY
CROSS-CULTURALLY

Our conceptions about medical modalities are not the only understandings we draw on in relation to health. When we try to fix something or to maintain it in good working order, many of our actions are guided by the way in which we think it—whether a relationship, a motorcycle, a pie, or a person—has been put together. Accordingly, health cultures everywhere entail, among other things, ideas about how the body works. While cross-cultural differences in these ideas are vast, bodies themselves are generally the same worldwide, and there are many underlying similarities in different cultures' anatomical and physiological notions. Further, as women provide the majority of primary care, many basic ideas about the body may be **gynocentric**, or modeled on female caretakers' own bodies' functioning (Sobo 1993).

Not only do we share, as human beings, the same basic body form and structure worldwide, but we also live under the same laws of physics. Rivers blocked by logs or debris overflow their banks; rust stiffens or petrifies hinges; heat melts ice or causes other solids to soften; and cold temperatures cause liquids to coagulate. While the material aspect of these processes will differ cross-culturally (e.g., for the Arctic Inuit the melting item might be snow; for the West Indian without a freezer it might be asphalt or fruit softening in the sun), the basic principles evinced will be the same. The basic principles also provide a framework for metaphorical elaboration. Many aspects of cross-cultural understandings about the body are simply elaborate abstractions of these basic principles, or selective but honest descriptions of basic, universal, embodied experiences (Lakoff 1987; Johnson 1987).

Human beings are creative. In addition to building on basic-level models to create explanatory systems, people exposed to different technologies will use different metaphors from these technologies to describe and understand body functions. Emily Martin demonstrates this in relation to the historical changes our own society has undergone: With industrialization, the body was increasingly imaged as a factory, converting energy into products (1987, 36–37). Importantly, like the factory—indeed like our society in general (government provides a good illustration)—the body was seen as hierarchically organized rather than as made up of systems that functioned as a committee of equals, each exerting mutual influence. More recently, computer-related and complex information management imagery has come into play.

THE INNER BODY

Most people worldwide have not spent much time exploring the inner cavities of the body. But common sense tells us that the torso contains at least one large cavity. Sometimes, there are a number of large cavities connected by pipes or tubes. Traditional Jamaicans, for example, view the trunk as divided into two spaces: the chest, and the belly, which extends from just under the breast to the groin.

Societies that slaughter animals for food and so regularly have direct dealings with their viscera (or who have ancestors who did) might envisage the cavities as full of sacs or bags. Traditional Jamaicans do: The belly, for example, holds air sacs (lungs), a urine bag (bladder), and, in women, a baby bag (womb).

FLOW, BLOCKAGE, AND CLEANLINESS

Elaborations on a basic spatial, hydraulic model that emphasizes flow and balance and incorporates container and conduit imagery, which Sobo (1993) calls a "flow model," can be found in ethnographic descriptions of a range of cultures. They are commonly invoked in lay explanations of menstruation; they are also a common and important part of indigenous theories of contraception or abortion and fertility enhancement. Flow models are described, for example, for the Amazonian Mehinaku (Gregor 1985, Chapter 5), for the Hua of New Guinea (Meigs 1983), and for biomedical scientists (Martin 1987, Chapter 3). Traditional Mexican ideas about *empacho*, in which digestion is blocked and food adheres to intestines or the stomach wall where it grows moldy, also indicate a flow model (Young and Garro 1982, 1459; Stafford 1978, 16).

In a flow system, it is essential that nothing block the body's pipes or tubes. To ensure that this does not happen, and for alleviation if it does, people can take occasional purges, as with laxatives. If left unattended, waste can build up behind blockages and fester, turning septic; blockages themselves can rot, releasing toxins into the system. In the United Kingdom, many traditionally feared "the dangers of constipation," which include the release of impurities into the bloodstream (Helman 2007, 31). Some referred to this process as "autointoxication" (Payer 1996, 116). These theories and beliefs help to explain the therapies adopted, which include treatments such as purging with enemas or medicines to reestablish or maintain the flow. Even if such therapy does not make biomedical sense (and sometimes it does), it makes cultural sense, following a logic for which culture provides the basis.

Purges in many cultures are meant to cleanse all bodily systems, including the circulatory system, urinary system, and respiratory system. The medicines that affect these internal cleanings can, but need not, be specialized; for many, bodily systems are interconnected and drainage is through the bottom parts, so waste from all of them might be excreted in feces or flushed out on urination. Similarly, vomiting (whether induced or naturally occurring) might serve this purpose.

Likewise, poisons may be drawn out through the skin, as with poultices (facial masks, popular with some American women, work this way) or through cupping or coin rubbing. The latter therapy, associated with Asian cultures, involves rubbing a coin on the skin to "draw out" the illness. In cupping, a heated cup is placed on the skin, creating a vacuum. As with coin rubbing, cupping can leave raised red welts.

People often use coin rubbing on children. The welts might suggest intentional child abuse. It is essential to realize that this is not the case, but that coin rubbing is done as a demonstration of love and caring (Korbin 1987, 28). The following case demonstrates:

> A Vietnamese girl named Kathy Dinh was in her first year at an American elementary school. She was not feeling very well one morning so her mother rubbed the back of her neck with a coin. She then felt well enough to attend school. Later in the day, however, she began to feel worse and went to see the school nurse. When the nurse discovered the welts on Kathy's neck, she immediately assumed she was seeing a case of child abuse and conscientiously reported the Dinhs to the authorities. The situation was finally straightened out, but it created a great deal of needless embarrassment for Kathy's family.
>
> (Galanti 2008, 198)

KEEPING EQUILIBRIUM

Not all cultures are so focused on keeping the internal body clean, or flow unimpeded. But most do have some notion of equilibrium, and strive to maintain some sort of balance. Even biomedical practitioners talk often of balance: Hormone imbalances, vitamin deficiencies, bacterial imbalances in the gut, and many other problems are conceptualized in terms of an equilibrium model of health.

HOT AND COLD

In many Latin American and Caribbean traditions and in some others, maintaining a balance between hot and cold is essential. Illness happens when the body (which generally is self-regulating) becomes too cool or too hot. For instance, among many Latin Americans and Caribbeans, menstruation and childbirth both are hot states. The body heats up and expels either menstrual blood or a baby. A hot body is open or vulnerable to the penetration of cold and other forces in a way that the body ordinarily would not be. Dangerous exposure must be avoided.

To this end, postpartum Puerto Ricans in one U.S. study reported avoiding cold foods. Ingestion of such foods would lead their postpartum discharges to clot and solidify, perhaps leading the waste in the discharge to be reabsorbed into the body rather than running out. This could cause nervousness or madness. To offset this threat, the women drank tonics containing garlic, chocolate, cinnamon, and other foods classified as hot (Snow and Johnson 1988, as cited in Helman 1995, 22; such practices still are common).

In some contexts, rather than to counterbalance disequilibrium, treatments seek to further heat or cool the body. For example, if the body is heating up in order to expel some toxin, further heating might help the body accomplish this task, thereby speeding recovery.

Importantly, although sick bodies do feel hot and cold, hot and cold are not necessarily thermal designations but rather symbolic constructions concerning the essential character of an item or state. As one early ethnographic report showed, classification may be based on color (or darkness or lightness), gender associations (maleness or femaleness), origin (e.g., foods from the sea or grown underground are cold while foods grown in direct sunlight are hot), and nutritive value (often, foods seen as supernutritious are hot) (Logan 1977). Sometimes the designation of a food, substance, or act as hot or cold is an after-the-fact justification of empirically observed bodily effects (Foster 1994, 75).

BODY FLUIDS

Sometimes, thermal systems are balanced around not only heat and coolness but also dryness and wetness, and specific body fluids can be involved. In French medicine, the liver and its bile are central (Payer 1996). In African Caribbean as well as in African American medicine, blood is key.

In an early example of case study writing demonstrating the necessity of what has come to be called cultural competence or sensitivity—and one that still has currency today—Korbin and Johnston (1982) describe a conflict over blood testing in a pediatric hospital that pitted a mother from Belize against a staff of biomedical clinicians. The mother felt that clinicians were harming her sick daughter with diagnostic blood tests, which she felt were needless. She was concerned about the loss of blood, and the disequilibrium in her small daughter's already weak body that was bound to happen if blood drawing did not stop. Accused of "ignorance" as well as "child abuse," and threatened with legal action, the mother resorted to bringing her daughter herbal teas, to " 'build her blood back up' " (261).

It is worth mentioning that in addition to her worries about blood depletion, the mother feared that hospital staff members were drawing excess quantities of blood so that they could sell it for a profit. Such worries do trace back to real-life situations in which similar wrongdoings have occurred; a blood-trafficking ring was in fact broken up just a few years after this girl's case (Blumenthal 1988). Today, trafficking in the United States includes organs as well (Dowling 2009).

Sometimes, when people use the word "blood," they refer to something altogether different, and this issue is quite relevant in the context of health care provision. For Caribbean peoples, for example, blood comes in two types: white and red. When unqualified by adjective or context, the word "blood" in Jamaica means the red kind, built from thick, dark liquid items such as red bean soup, English-style stout, or red-colored edibles such as tomatoes.

"Sinews," another form of blood, comes from okra, fish eyes, and other light-colored gelatinous foods, such as egg whites. Overexposure to the sun or excess tiring work can dry it out. Sinews include, but is not limited to, synovial fluid, which does resemble egg whites and lubricates the joints. The eyes are filled with sinews and glide in their sockets with its aid. Sinews is also associated with the nerves and with procreation. Many call it "white" blood in comparison to the red. Both kinds of blood are essential for good health.

Because the blood is so important, its qualities must be monitored. Not only must it be kept clean and thermally regulated, but it also must be neither too thick nor too thin, too bitter nor too sweet, too high nor too low in the body.

BALANCE IN ACCUMULATING SYSTEMS

Worldwide, a number of societies have developed highly sophisticated equilibrium-based systems of health by elaborating on the basic idea of bodily balance so that many body components and many types of qualities are implicated. These systems, generically called **humoral systems** because they all involve humors or body substances, refer not only to the physiological workings of the human body but also to social interactions and to cosmological concepts and nonorganic elements as well. As Leslie explained more than 30 years ago, "The arrangement and balance of elements in the human body were microcosmic versions of their arrangement in society at large and throughout the universe" (1976, 4). Factors such as sex, age, the season, diet, activities, and the tenor of one's relationships influence a person's equilibrium.

Classic humoral medicine, or Galenic medicine, stems from Hippocratic medicine (after the Greek theorist Hippocrates, 460 BC). The Greek physician Galen systematized and adapted the Hippocratic teachings into the Galenic system, which dominated in Europe until the germ theory of the late 1900s changed the direction of scientific medical investigation (Magner 1992, 93).

Galenic medicine teaches that the body contains four liquids or humors: blood, phlegm (mucus), yellow bile (stomach secretions, as in vomit), and black bile (according to Foster, possibly fecal matter darkened by blood; 1994, 5). Each humor has hot or cold and wet or dry properties, and each is associated with a "complexion" or temperament: sanguine (cheerful), phlegmatic (lethargic or unemotional), bilious or choleric (quick-tempered), and melancholic (sad). Further associations were made between humors and basic elements (accordingly, four were identified: wind or air, water, fire, and earth), as well as with the four seasons. As long as the four humors are in balance, health ensues. Imbalance can be treated by removing excesses, as by purging or vomiting, or by correcting for deficiencies that can be made up through special diets.

Knowledge of Galenic medicine gradually diffused eastward. The system diffused was called **Tibb-i-Yunani** in Arabic, or **Unani**, which means Greek medicine (Foster 1994, 13; Leslie 1976, 2). Today, many Islamic people maintain hot-cold distinctions, base their diet on Unanic precepts, and even divide all drugs according to these qualities.

At the end of the seventh century, Muslims were moving westward, and Galenic medicine diffused to Spain and Portugal via northern Africa and then to Latin America (Foster 1994, 14). Foster argues that the most important roots of thermal equilibrium systems in Latin America stem from Europe. However, the universal experiential basis of hot-cold conceptualizations and notions of balance suggests that equilibrium models would have existed in Latin America and the Caribbean, even without colonialism, as locally generated variations on a universal theme. European knowledge was incorporated if suitable and useful and rejected if not.

Some Galenic teachings also were taken into the **Ayurvedic** system, a similarly complex system that dates back some 4,000 years and is now practiced mainly in North India, but also in Pakistan, Bangladesh, Sri Lanka, and throughout the Arab world (Gesler 1991, 16). In Ayurveda, there are only three humors (phlegm, bile, and wind or flatulence), but there are seven body components: blood, flesh, fat, bone, marrow, semen, and food juice. Five elements exist: Ether, which is like the atmosphere, is the fifth. As in Greek medicine, heat and coolness also are important, and balance ensures good health (Foster 1994, 8).

The same is true in traditional Chinese medicine. However, this system centers on two contrasting forces: *yin* and *yang*. Yin subsumes all that is dark, moist, watery, and female; yang is comprised of all that is light, dry, fiery, and male. The idea of specific humors—and in Chinese medicine there are six (Leslie 1976, 4)—seems to have been appended to an initial yin-yang matrix (Foster 1994, 11). In any case, each organ is associated with yin or yang, and sophisticated procedures such as acupuncture, whereby needles are inserted into particular spots on the body and manipulated, are used to free up or redirect the energy flow. A basic concept of this system is that of the vital life force, or *qi*. Each individual body is pervaded with this energy, which allows physical function and maintains health and vitality (Ergil 1996, 195).

Chinese medicine, used as early as 1500 BC, is still practiced in China, which for nearly 50 years has had an extensive national program of combining traditional and Western medicine as formal components of their health care system (Bodeker 1996, 281). It is also practiced in Chinese communities throughout the world.

Kleinman (1984) observed that despite their relative independence there have been various degrees of borrowing and modernization in all these systems; he sees this as "a sign of a living, changing tradition in contradistinction to an historical artifact" (148). That is, these traditions, like any traditions, are not monolithic and unitary, but are constantly undergoing change, as is biomedicine. Leslie reminds us, however, that these traditions "maintained their individual characters although they were in contact with each other. The integrity of the separate traditions needs to be emphasized" (1976, 2).

Although they were "relatively independent," these health traditions "evolved in similar ways," all becoming professional branches of scientific learning with professional standards for education and practice (Leslie 1976, 3). As with the biomedical profession, authority of practitioners in these accumulating systems is vested in highly respected texts, special ways of dressing, and ethical codes. The theoretical bases for these systems were also derived by the "scientific method," if we understand by that term logical reasoning and conclusions based upon observations of various phenomena. The concepts of balance, flow, energy, temperature, and so forth are not so foreign to biomedicine: After all, blood pressure readings measure blood flow; specialists talk of one's hormonal or electrolyte balance; thermoregulation is at stake in conditions like hypothermia; and fevers, measured with thermometers, indicate infections.

BODY SIZE AND SHAPE

Body concepts are not limited to physiology. Cultures also have ideals for body shape and size. One area that has lately received much attention is weight, reflecting our own culturally constructed concern over fatness. In her cross-cultural review on the topic, Cassidy (1991) found that socially dominant individuals with sound relationships are usually large (relatively speaking). Bigness tends to ensure reproductive success and survival in times of scarcity and, cross-culturally, plumpness is generally considered attractive.

Such is the case in many of the West African societies from which people were taken to the United States as slaves. In some of these societies' traditions, those who can afford to do so seclude their adolescent girls in special "fattening rooms" and, after a period of ritual education and heavy eating, the girls emerge fat, attractive, and nubile (Brink 1989).

In Jamaican tradition, where a respected adult is called a "big man" or a "big woman," good relations involve food sharing, and people on good terms with others are ideally large. Weight loss signals social neglect. A Jamaican seeing someone grow thin might wonder about the sorts of life stresses that have caused the weight loss, rather than offering congratulations for it and attributing it to a "good" diet, as many middle- and upper-class Americans do without reflection. U.S. residents living in our inner cities, on the other hand, also worry about weight loss among friends or relatives. Thinness might be a symptom of HIV infection or tuberculosis, it may indicate that a person is addicted to crack cocaine or other dangerous substances, or it may simply signify poverty.

In the United States, being overweight is generally associated with unattractiveness, and internalization of this stigma (even by those who are not fat) has been connected with eating disorders—specifically anorexia nervosa and bulimia. A fat body may be seen as signifying "moral laxity" or a lack of self-control, which can lead to discrimination in employment (Bordo 1993; Wolf 1991, 179–217).

Ironically, as our population is getting fatter, some are experiencing even more job discrimination, increasing their chances of being impoverished and further affecting their health. For instance, between 1981 and 2000, the fat-linked "wage penalty" nearly doubled for women. In 1981, a woman in the 75th percentile for BMI or body mass index (e.g., 5'4" tall and 165 pounds) earned 4.3 percent less than a woman in the 25th percentile (5'4" tall and 120 pounds); in 2000, the difference was 7.5 percent. White women are particularly vulnerable to such bias (Lempert 2007). Social-structural factors as well as cultural differences are at play.

SEXUAL BIOLOGY: AN OBJECTIVE SCIENCE?

The conceptualization of male and female bodies also differs from society to society—geographically as well as historically. For example, while mainstream medicine presently views male and female bodies as two distinct entities, Thomas Laqueur (1990) has shown that sexual difference was, until recently, a matter of degree and not kind among many Europeans. "Language marks this view of sexual difference," he says. "For two millennia the ovary, an organ that by the early nineteenth century had become a synecdoche for woman, had not even a name of its own. Galen refers to it with the same word he uses for the male testes" (4–5). A synecdoche is a metaphor in which a part (ovary) stands for a whole (woman). Because men and women were viewed as basically more anatomically similar than distinct prior to the latter 1700s, male genitalia could be understood as merely the external expression of what in females was retained in the internal area of the groin. The penis, for example, was understood as an extruded vagina (Laqueur 1990).

But for various reasons, in the eighteenth century, a belief in fundamental differences replaced the belief in congruity between the sexes. This led anatomists to focus not on similarities but on distinctions between the male and female body. A vast amount of data demonstrating no difference between male and female anatomy and physiology, such as the fact that male and female reproductive organs share common developmental origins from the fetal stage, was ignored or treated as if absent while differences in form and function were highlighted.

Biology is not, then, so objective. The body is not the unmovable ground that we like to think it is. Culture determines, to some degree, the size and shape we see as natural, and what we find when we peer inside the body. What explains the cultural shift in ways of seeing the body that led from the one-sex to the two-sex model? As Laqueur explains, after the French Revolution, custom lost its force: The new egalitarianism threatened to undermine men's superordinate position. So the gender status quo was justified by grounding female inferiority and subordination in her distinct biological makeup. Biology became destiny. Laqueur (1990) thus demonstrates that biology and medicine are culturally influenced fields that can serve to underpin dominant ideologies. In A. Young's words, "medical practices are simultaneously ideological practices" (1982, 271).

BODY, MIND, AND SOCIETY

Health cultures are not concerned solely with the body corporeal (Frankenberg's term; 1994, 1326). They also entail ideas about the mind or the conscious, interactive self and ways to keep it in good working condition. Some of these concern good living—conducting oneself in keeping with the recommended social and moral order. For example, maintaining good interpersonal relations limits one's exposure to strong emotions, which might affect the mind, and to the wrath of others, which might be vented on one's health. Such relations may include those with kin, friends, and neighbors, as well as deceased relatives or other spiritual entities.

Improper treatment of the corporeal or physical body also can affect the mind, just as mind trouble can manifest itself in the corporeal body. So treatment of the mind may involve treatment of the body, and vice versa. In fact, these two dimensions of experience— mental and physical—are inextricably interconnected despite the Western tendency to dichotomize or bisect them. This is changing, especially with the recognition by biomedicine that stress contributes to physical responses such as high blood pressure, heart disease, and physical distress and symptoms. And yet, biomedical doctors may treat nervousness with medications designed to alter brain chemistry. Traditional Jamaicans also focus treatments for nervousness on the body, prescribing certain remedies and food supplements meant to strengthen the physical nerves and restore a certain kind of "white" blood, the lack of which contributes to nerve problems (Sobo 1996b).

But in certain Latin American traditions, the symptoms of nerves may be attributed ultimately to soul loss (literally, loss of the soul), and ritual as well as physical action will need to be taken. The physical processes immediately underlying a condition, sometimes called the immediate or **proximate** cause, is not as important as the **ultimate** cause—the reason why that problem is bothering that individual at that point in time. Indeed, physical processes might not even be implicated at all in particular forms of suffering or distress. This demonstrates the necessity of a broad conceptualization of health; most health systems worldwide involve and address far more than simple physical problems when restoring or promoting good health.

SEEKING HEALTH

RECOGNIZING SYMPTOMS

It is quite possible to be ill without being diseased. Likewise, it is possible to have a disease without being ill. Illness is not merely a person's reaction to a disease. Indeed, it is not disease that spurs a person to seek medical treatment but rather it is his or her "experience of suffering which engenders the whole medical enterprise. The sufferer's judgment rather than that of biomedicine defines the *underlying problem*" (Hahn 1984, 17, emphasis in original; also see Mechanic 1962).

The underlying problem, or sickness, according to Hahn, "is a matter of unwanted conditions of self" (1995, 22). And while certain conditions will be universally unwanted, "what is major sickness for one may be a minor irritation for another" (23); a sore knee will merely bother the academic but will be cause for great alarm in the Olympic athlete. Unwanted conditions of self vary not only from individual to individual but also from culture to culture: "The good Buddhist pursues experiences of generalized hopelessness for which the Westerner seeks treatment" (Hahn 1995, 35).

The recognition of symptoms, the first step in what Chrisman has famously termed "the health seeking process," depends on cultural definitions of normal health, as well as understandings about the causes and contexts of sickness (1977). Some of the important factors here are symptom visibility and frequency. The visibility and frequency of the symptom in question in others and the way this compares to its visibility and frequency in one's own case is key, for the former provides a context for evaluating the significance of the latter. Also taken into account is the level of danger to life and interference with lifestyle and activities of daily living, or impairment, that the symptoms or the syndrome entailed portend.

Chrisman's inclusion of the degree to which the individual thinks that something can be done is also a part of the **Health Belief Model**, a theoretical framework for predicting the likelihood for care seeking (Rosenstock 1966; also see Becker 1974). This model, a health psychology mainstay, posits that an individual's subjective evaluation of an illness situation, including the value placed on a particular outcome and the belief that a particular action will result in that outcome, is the key variable in decisions regarding behavior change or the use of particular health services. The patient's "common sense" may conflict with a public health recommendation or clinical judgment (see Becker and Maiman 1975).

As noted by Cockerham (2010), the Health Belief Model has limited applicability: It applies only to voluntary, preventive care seeking. It does not address those individuals who seek care based primarily on the clarity and severity of symptoms. Cockerham further notes that individuals often do not take action unless they think "that being ill will result in serious difficulty. Thus, the individual's subjective assessment of the health situation becomes the critical variable in the utilization of health services" (132).

Also relevant here is the fact that many people who are diseased do not perceive themselves as ill, and vice versa. Because in most instances disease is **self-limiting** (e.g., a bout of flu generally ends even without medical treatment), this is not necessarily a bad thing. However, it may pose a problem for biomedical treatment regimens when no disease is found, and a problem for society when those who are sick get sicker or pass their disease to others.

In addition to being self-defined, ill health can be other-defined, in which case others perceive an individual's symptoms, define them as an illness condition, and then call the illness to the individual's attention (Mechanic 1978). Although the biomedical system is organized so that individual patients present their own cases, in reality many people are assisted by others when it comes to identifying and interpreting symptoms and weighing treatment options.

In any case, once symptoms are recognized, individuals may adopt a culturally prescribed **sick role**. The sick role, a concept introduced in 1951 by Talcott Parsons, legitimizes sickness under four conditions: The individual who is sick is exempt from "normal" social roles, is not at fault or responsible for the sickness condition, should try to get well, and should seek technically competent help and co-operate with the physician. Thus the *physician* becomes an agent of social control, and help seeking elsewhere is not "legitimate."

The narrow bounds of legitimacy in this model, its middle-class orientation, postulations of role exemption and individual responsibility, definition of "technically competent help," and failure to address the variability of individuals and social groups have been criticized as biomedically biased and culturally limiting (Mechanic 1962; Gordon 1966; Twaddle 1969). However, the concept of the sick role continues to contribute to an understanding of the desirability of health for any culture, however defined. In addition, because many types of deviant behavior, such as overeating, drug addiction, and smoking, can endanger the public's health, medicine acts as an agent of social control under the auspices of the state. The sick role thus contributes to an understanding of the mechanisms of social stability (Turner 1984).

There are numerous other explanatory models and theories of illness perception (e.g., Suchman 1965; Freidson 1960), most of which have a number of similarities to those we have presented (i.e., Chrisman 1977; Hahn 1984, 1995; Mechanic 1978; Parsons 1951). All have some limitations; for example, many focus on symptom perception and the consequent decision to visit a physician. But symptoms are not always grouped together in the same way cross-culturally, other aspects of illness can drive people to consult healers, and the physician is not always the first or even last choice of provider. Other limitations include the assumption that seeking biomedical care is *the* legitimate response to illness. But there are many other paths to health.

PATTERNS OF RESORT

By 1980, we knew that only 6 to 30 percent of medical problems were ever brought to the attention of a biomedical clinician (Demers et al. 1980). Even when study participants were covered for free biomedical treatments by prepaid medical insurance, most care was procured within the household. In about one-quarter of cases, no action was taken. In another one-quarter, "home remedies" were used. More often, people self-medicated with over-the-counter preparations or prescription drugs left over from another occasion (1088).

The concept of biomedically oriented "lay-referral" refers to the fact that when people become ill, they first turn to family and friends, then to suggested lay "experts," and finally, if nothing works, to a physician and the biomedical system, although lay norms may influence this option (Freidson 1960). This behavior is consistent with Romanucci-Ross's **hierarchy of resort** (1977 [1969]). However, while Romanucci-Ross was concerned with acculturation issues, that phrase today generally means that people try the most familiar or simplest and cheapest treatment first and then seek more expensive, complex, or unfamiliar treatments if necessary.

While treatment choice can follow a hierarchical sequence, often patterns of resort are cumulative and pluralistic, involving many treatment modalities at once. And people do not necessarily comply with all the rules surrounding each type of treatment. People often creatively combine recommendations, coming up with the regimen they feel is right for them. As Chrisman (1977) has pointed out, the "health seeking process" is dynamic, and people are constantly reevaluating their symptoms and actions and revising their plans.

COMPLEMENTARY AND ALTERNATIVE APPROACHES

In many cases, people who seek biomedical assistance already have used some type of home treatment. Snow cites a Michigan study in which 78 percent of 50 elderly individuals being treated biomedically for hypertension had used home remedies in the past six months (1993, 128–29).

In recent years, home remedies have been subsumed in a larger category, **complementary and alternative medicine** or CAM. CAM medical practices are neither routinely taught in U.S. medical schools nor routinely paid for by regular health insurance policies. Technically speaking, complementary medicine is used *with* biomedicine; alternative medicine is used *in place of* it. Nonetheless, many people use the terms interchangeably or simply say "CAM." And, however termed, millions of Americans use these approaches after defining themselves as ill.

To biomedical practitioners, the frequency of CAM use may not be obvious. A recent review of the literature done in conjunction with a study of pediatric CAM use, which includes consultation with CAM providers as well as home remedy use, reported that about only 40 percent of adult patients in the United States disclose CAM use to their physicians (Prussing et al. 2004). In regard to children, although three-quarters of pediatricians believe parents share CAM use with them, only perhaps one-quarter of parents say that they do. Earlier, a national study reported that 89 percent of those using other therapies did so without their doctors' recommendation or knowledge (Eisenberg et al. 1993, 249).

In this groundbreaking nationwide study, Eisenberg and colleagues (1993) found that one in three people used at least one "unconventional" (nonbiomedical) therapy in the past year. While prior studies often were limited to "home remedies," the term "unconventional therapy" in this study covered many relatively expensive therapies that people cannot carry out at home, such as chiropractic and acupuncture, in addition to herbal medicine and such. The number of visits recorded by Eisenberg's group, 425 million, exceeded the 388 million visits to all primary care physicians in 1990. Significantly more people aged 25–49 used unconventional therapies than those who were older or younger.

More recent studies indicate the same if not more so: By 2007, nearly 40 percent of adults were using CAM. By that year, data on child's use was also being collected, and the pediatric figure in 2007 was 12 percent (P. Barnes, Bloom, and Nahin 2008). CAM use was higher among women and the more highly educated as well as those with higher incomes. The highest use was among people aged 30–70 (this differs from the earlier Eisenberg et al. findings, but may reflect simply the aging of Eisenberg et al.'s cohort). In terms of ethnic group, CAM use in 2007 was highest by far among Native Americans, one-half of whom used it, and lowest among African Americans and Hispanic Americans (about one-quarter of whom used it). What to make of the ethnic differences is unclear. It may be that the survey wording introduced unintended bias so that certain types of CAM more popular among some groups were uncounted; or, real differences may be reflected.

Of health problems treated by CAM, musculoskeletal problems have been the most common ones reported (P. Barnes, Bloom, and Nahin 2007). CAM has also been used to enhance developmental potential in children with Down syndrome (Prussing et al. 2004).

Psychologists Furnham and Beard (1995) found that people visit complementary medical practitioners because they believe more strongly that mental, emotional, and environmental factors play a significant part in both health and illness. They also tend to emphasize the importance of positive attitudes and happiness and take more control of their own health behavior (e.g., self-medication). Further, they do not tend to "blame the victim" for their own fate. But it remains unclear whether health beliefs lead people to choose CAM practitioners, or practitioners educate or lead patients to particular health beliefs; Furnham and Beard conclude it is probably a bit of both (1431).

Biomedicine has come to acknowledge the legitimacy of various CAM modalities. The National Institutes of Health created the National Center for Complementary and Alternative Medicine in 1998, expanding and enhancing what was the Office of Alternative Medicine, itself founded in 1992 in response to the need to learn more about CAM practices. By 1998, 8.6 percent of U.S. hospitals practiced at least some **integrative medicine**: They offered some complementary therapies along with biomedical ones. By 2004, the proportion had increased to almost 20 percent and another 24 percent of hospitals planned to add an integrative component in the future (Kam 2006) (see also Chapter 5).

THE MODALITIES: ETIOLOGICAL UNDERPINNINGS

THEORETICAL FRAMEWORKS OF VARIOUS SYSTEMS

In diagnosing and treating illness, it is sometimes important to know how the body normally functions and how, in sickness, those processes have been physiologically impeded. For example, the Pennsylvania Dutch, who have descended from German immigrants who settled in various areas of Pennsylvania, generally rely on **homeopathic** treatments. In homeopathy, the remedy, if used on a healthy person, would produce the same symptoms as those exhibited by the sick individual. This is not a unique concept; it is also used biomedically in treating allergies and in using live or dead viruses in minute amounts to stimulate the body's immune reactions.

At other times, mental and social processes are deemed more important than physiological ones for isolating causes and devising treatment strategies. Family therapists, for example, treat whole family units as systems that may have encouraged the presence of sickness (e.g., anorexia, alcoholism) in one member. Families are then taught to think in new ways, and to adopt different social interactions. Similarly, some shamans or diviners might treat illness by prescribing a confession and atonement session in which family members confess or declare wrongdoings to others and try to set their relationships right (e.g., Janzen 1978).

The latter kind of treatment, which centers on social relations, is called "personalistic." A modality such as homeopathy, in which individual biological pathologies are treated, is called "naturalistic."

Naturalistic treatment also can be addressed to illness brought about by strong emotions when these induce an internal, impersonal imbalance in the body. The **naturalistic-personalistic** scheme, which we discuss in more detail later, was offered by George Foster in the context of a cross-cultural examination of disease etiologies (theories of disease origins) in 1976. It does not take structural factors into account.

Another simple, two-part (and likewise structurally naive) etiological model holds that illness can stem from the bodily intrusion or extrusion of substances, essences, or objects. The intrusion-extrusion model we describe is adapted from and builds on early classification schemes (e.g., Clements 1932). Extrusion-caused illness can occur as a result of soul loss or the loss of blood or nonabsorption of nutrients, as with diarrhea. In intrusion-caused illnesses, noxious substances such as poisons, germs, or evil spirits penetrate the body's barriers, disturbing its internal balance. In this model, illness due to a bleeding wound or to the loss of one's soul are classed together as extrusive, just as germs and evil spirits are similarly categorized as intrusive. However, treatment for germ-caused or spirit-caused illness does differ, and this is what Foster was getting at with his 1976 naturalistic-personalistic typology.

Around the same time, Young described another two-part scheme in which illness was seen either as **internalized** or **externalized**. Internalizing systems, says Young, focus on physiological explanations or mechanisms, and on the "biophysical signs which mark the course of disease episodes" (1986 [1976], 140). Illness is encapsulated in the individual body. Biomedicine would be a good example of an internalizing system.

Externalizing systems, on the other hand, ascribe more importance to events that happen outside of the body that is sick. In these systems, "pathogenic agencies are usually purposive and often human or anthropomorphized [i.e., conceptualized in human form]. Diagnostic interests concentrate on discovering what events could have brought the sick person to the attention of the pathogenic agency" (Young 1986 [1976], 141). Externalizing systems are more concerned with ultimate causes than with proximate internal mechanisms. The Navajo practice of having a specialist sing, bringing the ill person's world back into balance and thereby treating the root of his or her disorder, is part of an externalizing system (Adair, Deuschle, and Barnett 1988, 7, 170)

While there are subtle differences between the two schemes, the naturalistic-personalistic and internalizing-externalizing schemes in many ways overlap. Whether one or the other is invoked depends on the aspects of illness that the theorist seeks to highlight or explain.

SOCIAL COMPLEXITY, CULTURAL UNITY, AND CHANGING MEDICAL SYSTEMS

Young (1986 [1976]) offers some important suggestions about the evolution of health systems using the externalizing-internalizing model. Young holds that internalizing systems evolved from externalizing systems in societies that grew complex, as happened in the United States with modernization and industrialization.

Externalizing systems focus on social and cosmological relations. They are interlinked with other cultural domains, such as religion, and have little conceptual autonomy (Young 1986 [1976]).

But internalizing systems are autonomous to a high degree. That is, physical health is not overtly linked to social or moral health. Young explains this as stemming from a division of labor. In small-scale societies, the division of labor is low, and there is not much specialization; according to Young (1986 [1976]) this explains the overlap between healing and other cultural domains (e.g., legal, religious, etc.).

In large-scale societies, we find complex patterns of labor division. The conceptual autonomy of internalizing schemes is, Young (1986 [1976]) says, linked to the emergence of specialization and extreme distinction between cultural domains, which comes with such complex patterns. In large-scale societies, where cultural realms are fragmented, internalizing medicines, which focus on the body and pay little attention to legal, religious, and other dimensions of life, can evolve.

In biomedicine, as in all internalizing systems, religion and magic have limited explanatory power; curers need no supernatural abilities. Health is, in theory, segmented off from other aspects of culture, such as religion, and social relationships. Biomedicine even generally divorces mind from body, with different branches specializing in physical or mental health.

NATURALISTIC APPROACHES

While the externalizing-internalizing scheme is, in some contexts, quite useful, we find that the naturalistic-personalistic model has more immediate or practical utility. The rest of the chapter examines the model in detail, and uses it to organize the presentation of practitioner types.

Naturalistic models explain sickness as being due to impersonal forces or conditions, including "cold, heat, winds, dampness, and, above all, by an upset in the balance of the basic body elements" (Foster 1976, 775). Foster explains that all naturalistic modalities are based on ideas of equilibrium. The humoral systems described earlier in this chapter are good examples and so is biomedicine, which views illness as a disruption of function at a physiological level. Causes of such a disruption may include attack by viruses and bacteria, breakdown of biological systems, and so on. Viewed naturalistically, illness can be treated without social, supernatural, or spiritual intervention.

Cross-culturally, five types of naturalistic practitioners exist: herbalists, chemists, surgeons, bodyworkers, and lay midwives (we will use the term "midwife" to indicate lay midwives, as opposed to midwives in the nursing profession). The inclusion of the midwife may seem strange, because this category of healer is determined by the body system or event attended to, rather than by a method of healing per se (e.g., with herbs, or chemicals, or by cutting, or manipulating). Moreover, pregnancy is generally not defined cross-culturally as an illness to be healed; it was not considered so historically (see Eastman and Loustaunau 1987). Indeed, in various states, including New Mexico, midwives were not categorized as health care providers and thus were not subject to medical licensure until the 1920s. But midwifery is an extremely common occupation cross-culturally, with the purpose of providing care and assistance to preserve the health of the mother, and so we include it in our list (see Table 4.2).

The skills categories described here are not mutually exclusive; while in some cultures practitioners are extremely specialized, in others there may be a significant amount of overlap. Humoral doctors, for example, may be both chemists and herbalists. There may also be

Table 4.2
Practitioners

Naturalistic Practitioners	Personalistic Practitioners	
Herbalists	**Magical**	**Religious**
Chemists	• Healers	• Priests
Surgeons	• Sorcerers	• Shamans
Bodyworkers		
Midwives		

overlap in medical systems themselves; for example, biomedical and Ayurvedic approaches are used in combination by many practitioners in India where medical **syncretism** or the active aggregation or blending of these two systems has a long history. The degree of overlap will differ from culture to culture, possibly influenced by social complexity and the specialization entailed in it, much as described earlier in relation to the development of internalizing systems.

The distribution of the five types of skills across the sectors of health care and the degree of status attributed to them also will differ from culture to culture. However, skills that involve longer periods of training and the use of controlled substances or materials, or expensive, specialized technological devices with limited availability, are most likely to be confined to practitioners in Kleinman's (1986a) professional sector. Those skills involving everyday knowledge and locally available resources are likely to be used in the household production of health (Kleinman's popular sector [1986a]). Where technology is idealized, those practitioners with technological skills may be vested with more authority than those who work with low-tech or no devices.

Herbalists treat people with or prescribe curative and preventive medicines made from plants. While many of the plants used can be classed as herbs, other plants, roots, bark, and other substances also may be made use of. Various plant parts can be prepared as teas or infusions to be drunk, or they can be kept in suspension in bottles of oil or alcohol, which will absorb various elements from them, and then can be used in small doses. Plants also might be ground down and mixed into pastes for external application. Some plants or plant combinations are smoked or absorbed through various body orifices, such as the nose.

A wide variety of foods are derived from plants, and so some practitioners classed as herbalists may make dietary recommendations. For example, the Jamaican condition called *nerves*, which comes about when a person's vital supply of *sinews*, a type of white blood, is depleted, can be treated with food supplements, as noted earlier. A diet rich in okra and other slimy foods as well as liquidous foods light in color is recommended.

While herbalists generally focus on plants, occasionally they may make recommendations related to nonplant foods. Herbalists also occasionally use minerals or other elements in their medicines, including vitamin supplements or maybe aspirin (derived from willow bark), but generally they do not use manufactured or isolated chemical compounds. Plants themselves and the ways they are used, rather than the isolated chemical compounds in them, are thought to be what effects a cure (see Etkin 1990).

Medicines made from isolated chemical elements are the domain of the **chemist** (this term is used in the United Kingdom to denote pharmacists). Chemists may rely on products that can be purchased over the counter to make their medicines or treatment recommendations; they also can, in some cases, prescribe controlled substances, as through a pharmacy (but not in a U.S. pharmacy, where unrestricted independent diagnosing and prescribing are prohibited).

In certain economically poorer nations, we find chemists specializing in injections. Often the substance injected is a vitamin compound. The **injectionist** means to promote health but unfortunately often reuses unsterile needles, which is implicated in the spread of HIV and other pathogens.

Another category of naturalistic practitioner is the **surgeon**, who cuts into the body to mend or alter it. Sometimes, a surgeon removes offending or diseased organs or substances from the body's inner reaches. Other times, the surgeon cuts into the surface organs, as for blood letting or removing warts. While much surgery is corrective, other times it is preventive: Male circumcision, for example, is thought by biomedical specialists to protect men against penile infection and women against cervical cancer; it also protects against HIV infection (see Chapter 8). In certain regions of Africa, surgeons remove milk teeth as a preventive measure should a child be infected with tetanus or lockjaw; if this should happen, an oral portal will be open so that nutrition can be taken (Kate Hill, personal communication).

The **bodyworker,** or the musculo-skeletal specialist, manipulates the body to restore health. The category includes people who specialize in massage, bone setting, and skeletal realignment. The chiropractor, who is concerned with the latter, comes under this heading, as does the osteopath, who is also a biomedical practitioner, and the physical therapist. The Mexican *sobador* is concerned with all the aspects of bodywork, and may also massage the nerves and "cool the blood" to reduce swelling and inflammation, soften muscle, and reduce pain and tension (Loustaunau 1990, 659).

The **midwife** works to bring about successful childbirth. The medicine midwives practice is primarily preventive and supportive and ensures, rather than restores, well-being. Generally, midwives are women who already have borne children of their own. Often, they learn their trade through a period of apprenticeship and may have specialized knowledge in all things related to reproduction, including abortion, contraception, and treatments for infertility. In some cultures, midwives may take care of male infant circumcisions as well.

In the United States, nurse midwives are distinguished from lay midwives. One category, both, or neither may be allowed to practice, depending upon state laws. Much depends upon the local medical profession's perception of the role of the midwife as related to biomedical practice (Eastman and Loustaunau 1987).

SPECIAL BLENDS

Practitioners of all five types work with the assumption that natural, pathophysiological bodily processes underlie the conditions they are treating. Sometimes, however, they may augment their naturalistic work with personalistic practices. So, in addition to the fact that both naturalistic and personalistic treatment practices can exist in one culture, one practitioner can draw on both types of technique.

Some midwives, for example, may execute ritual actions to ensure that evil spirits do not trouble their pregnant charges or new mothers, as in West Indian tradition. Sometimes this does happen, and midwives must drive the spirits away (or call in a personalistic specialist who can do so). In the United States, midwives often are seen as giving, in addition to naturalistic assistance, the personal and emotional support that is often absent in the biomedical approach to childbirth (Eastman and Loustaunau 1987). In recent years, more doctors have accepted midwife assistance, primarily from nurse midwives, and birthing centers give women more choices about having family present and in regard to how they want to have their babies.

The overt coexistence of both naturalistic and personalistic healing is evident in Jamaican tradition, where much medicine is naturalistic and sickness by default is seen as "natural." However, when a naturalistic treatment fails, or when sickness after sickness befalls a person, or when a condition just does not seem typical or normal, personalistic etiology may be traced. The coexistence of naturalistic and personalistic frameworks also is seen in the United States, with its officially naturalistic etiologies. Personalistic etiological notions are denigrated by the dominant culture, but nonetheless they are appealed to for answers that naturalistic etiological thought cannot provide: answers about the ultimate cause of sickness and suffering. As Irving Zola points out in relation to health surveys meant to determine how knowledgeable the public is about biomedical explanations,

We may be comforted by the scientific terminology if not the accuracy of [the respondent's] answers. Yet if we follow this questioning with the probe: "Why did you get X now?' or 'Of all the people in your community, family etc. who were exposed to X, why did you get ... ?", then the rational scientific veneer is pierced and the concern with personal and moral responsibility emerges quite strikingly. Indeed, the issue "why me?" becomes of great concern and is generally expressed in quite moral terms of what they did wrong.

(1972, 491; ellipsis in the original)

The "why me" question is as relevant today as it was when Zola wrote, and as it has been through the ages. For instance, a study was undertaken in Israel with mothers of children with Down syndrome caused, according to biomedicine, by the existence of an extra chromosome. When the mothers explained their unusual birth outcomes, none mentioned chromosomes, despite the fact that education levels in Israel are generally high and biomedicine is the dominant medical system there. Instead, they talked of the stress of the Arab-Israeli war, family quarrels, bad dreams, and the like (Chigier, as cited in Moore et al. 1980, 11; see also Prussing et al. 2005).

Even where naturalistic etiologies or internalizing systems predominate, some sicknesses, perhaps especially new or ill-understood diseases or those linked with private body parts, such as the anus, and ones associated with disfavored lifestyle choices such as smoking or using narcotics, will be construed as punishments. Indeed, as Foster (1976) points out in regard to naturalistic and personalistic etiologies, the two are not mutually exclusive, and although a people may favor one over the other in general, both ways of understanding sickness will be present.

The degree to which these personalistic beliefs intrude on naturalistic systems varies considerably, from just a little (a U.S. surgeon saying that, in the end, the success of an operation is in God's hands; the midwife who wears an amulet to guard against evil) to a lot. When the threshold to "a lot" has been crossed, then that practitioner would probably be classed as subscribing to a personalistic model of treatment. The question to be asked in determining a classification is, "To which model is primacy given?" And to be able to gauge this, a better understanding of the personalistic mode is needed.

However, any push to classify is inherently digressive. Because most traditions actually involve blends of both approaches, practitioners should try to meet patients' needs relating to both naturalistic and personalistic systems. One way to do this is by making sure to ask patients about concerns they may have regarding the downplayed dimension; for example, "What do you think is happening in your body?" or, in the case of the naturalistic practitioner, "Why do you think you caught it now?" (For more on this kind of clinical interviewing, see Chapter 7.) Being able to provide referrals, say to religious or spiritual specialists or to counselors, is important. No matter how well intended, an either-or position might be quite alienating. Even the staunchest supporter of biomedicine might need to have an answer "why" when a loved one dies of a disease that generally does not kill, or when someone who beat the odds of his or her condition last time succumbs this time around. It is extremely important for biomedical clinicians to have a basic understanding of these personalistic systems and beliefs.

PERSONALISTIC APPROACHES

In contrast to naturalistic modalities, where sickness is an impersonal condition related to impersonal forces, personalistic approaches posit the intervention or influence of an active external agent. The agent may be human (e.g., a sorcerer) or nonhuman (e.g., an ancestral ghost, an evil force, or a deity). Accident or chance cannot account for sickness here as it can in a naturalistic explanation; sickness is the result of an agent's purposive act.

Sometimes, a person will find her- or himself the victim of a witch or other agent who purposefully chooses him or her as a victim through malice. But often, the purposive acts are provoked by the individuals who find themselves sick. That is, they are retributional acts. The agent involved in retribution might be a neighbor, angered by some antisocial behavior, an ancestral ghost put out by a lack of attention to his or her memory, or a punishing god, angered by a moral infraction. This is how sin can lead to sickness (Sobo 1993).

In personalistic systems, writes Foster, emphasis is placed on "the need to make sure that one's social networks, with fellow human beings, with ancestors, and with deities, are maintained in good working order" (1976, 780). For, if not retribution, behavior that is out of order surely will provoke at least a warning, in the form of ill health, meant to push one back into line. People fear this and so try to behave; the fear of sickness, or anxiety over the possibility of punishment for breaking social and moral rules, serves as a mechanism for maintaining social order (Hallowell 1977 [1941], 132).

Landy suggests that this fear "assumes the greatest generalized importance in those social systems in which there are few or no institutionalized and formalized mechanisms for settling disputes and enforcing conformity" (1977, 132). In other words, illness anxiety is most likely to serve a positive social function in simple, small-scale societies—societies in which, as Lewis (1986) and Young (1986 [1976]) note, no specialization or segregation of cultural domains, such that health systems function independently, has occurred.

Personalistic therapies hinge on the determination of why sickness happens; diagnosis, which Foster (1976) explains is more important than treatment per se, involves asking "Why?" or "Who is responsible?" Once an agent is identified, treatment steps can be taken. These steps vary widely across sociocultural contexts, individual case situations, and often even between healers in the same context depending on the background and healing preferences of each. Despite variation, because ideas about the social and moral order are entailed, personalistic healing generally involves religious action. It may also or otherwise involve the practice of magic.

HEALING, MAGIC, AND RELIGION

Magic, as defined in Whiteford and Friedl (1992, 316), "is the attempt to manipulate the forces of nature to obtain certain results." Magic effects a supernatural pressure on nature so that things that would not normally happen, do. The action (e.g., burning garbage gathered from one's home and chanting a spell to reverse cancerous growth) leads directly to the result.

Religion, on the other hand, generally holds that there are forces more powerful than humans in the universe and that these higher powers—not humans—control certain outcomes, such as whether a cure will be effective on certain kinds of illnesses. So in religious healing we must persuade god(s), spirits, or spiritual forces to grant a certain result or instigate a particular chain of events on our behalf. Our action (e.g., doing good deeds and praying for Jesus to reverse cancerous growth) leads the higher or nonmortal powers to consider bringing about the result. Magic does; religion asks.

Religious action, by definition, entails the adoption of a moral stance that is pleasing to the higher power(s) and may involve magical rites (e.g., the Jewish practice of marking the doorpost with a mezuzah, or protective amulet; the Christian practice of reading the Bible aloud to rebuke evil spirits). When carried out in tandem with religious actions, magic is linked with ideas about a moral universe; however, it can be carried out in nonreligious contexts.

The principles behind **magical healing** (and **sorcery**, as magic is called when used for vengeance or malicious ends, such as causing sickness) are relatively straightforward and were famously described by Sir James Frazer. He called them, respectively, the law of similarity and the law of contact. Both are linked to the human capacity for symbolic thought (1942 [1922; first edition 1890]).

The *law of similarity* applies, for example, when sticking pins into a doll made to resemble an individual produces pain in that individual. It dictates that red medicine can be good for the blood or that leaves with spots might cure a rash. It can be applied by naturalistic healers as well as personalistic healers, and indeed it is. But the former see this as consistent with the laws of nature, not as bending or manipulating them, so although they may apply the law of similarity, they do not do so in a magical fashion.

The second principle of magic, the *law of contact*, generally guides people's choice of healing materials (once in contact, always in contact), as when a Jamaican healer known to Sobo treated the worn nightgown of a hospitalized woman with certain concoctions in order to make the woman herself well. It explains how the blood of Jesus can cure, or how a relic (a preserved piece of a saint's body) can have healing power. And it also explains why individuals from many cultures guard their body excretions or hair and nail clippings: Evil magic (sorcery) for retribution can be worked using these substances.

Religion, on the other hand, generally does not support vengeance against community members or kin (although that outcome still might happen). Treatment advised will benefit all by restoring social harmony while healing sick individuals. Because religious healing is concerned with issues of morality, many religions leave vengeance to the gods or other powerful forces. This is not to say that religious people never seek revenge or consult sorcerers—they do—but religious teachings may discourage intracommunity hate and destructive confrontations while encouraging reconciliation.

Just as there are two types of practitioners who heal using magic (magical healers and sorcerers), there are two types of religious healing specialists: the priest and the shaman. The **priest** undergoes formal training, and the power held resides in the office rather than the individual. The **shaman**, on the other hand, is powerful as an individual, and his or her power comes directly from the gods, spirits, or spiritual forces (Whiteford and Friedl 1992, 327). The priest can bring humans' messages or requests for healing, to the higher power(s), while the Shaman often brings the higher power(s) directly to the people, acting as a *medium* through which the power speaks, or as a *diviner* (328), revealing past actions connected with the illness event.

A priest praying with a hospitalized individual before an operation is helping him or her to ask for protection so that the surgeons, who are dealing only with the proximate or immediate cause of the illness and not the ultimate cause, which may be seen by the patient as having to do with sin or redemption, will get it right. Shamans, whose work generally is more dynamic, heal as instruments of the higher power(s). A faith healer who brings eyesight to the blind through the laying on of hands and chanting does so only because, in touching the blind individual, the healer serves a conduit for a god's or a spirit's or spiritual force's healing power. Faith healers, then, may be simply one type of shaman.

THE PLACEBO EFFECT

Personalistic healing can effect organic cures without affecting the proximate cause of an illness directly. This happens through the **placebo effect**. This effect is well utilized in many complementary therapeutics and is not unknown in biomedicine, where cures or improvements are effected with inert substances given to a patient who believes them to be medication. For example, as much as 50 percent of analgesic pain relief is due to a placebo response (Watkins 1996, 56).

Norman Cousins (1981 [1979], 56) has noted that in the United States a prescription for medication has a placebo effect. We view prescriptions as necessary because we live in a culture that focuses on drug therapy; every patient has been socialized to expect to leave a clinical setting with one, even if the physician deems it unnecessary; the prescription is a major part of the healing ritual. Pharmaceutical companies and advertisement also strongly promote prescription medications for a wide range of conditions that might be treated or controlled by alternative means. Patients have learned to demand pills and prescriptions, which generally are filled. If one doctor refuses, the patient will just keep searching for another who will comply with his wishes. "'Good medicine'," says Shorter, "bends in the wind of patient expectations" (1985, 235).

While placebos per se were often an overt part of medical practice in the past, physicians today are generally reluctant to use or even to discuss the use of the placebo; it is generally viewed as unethical and implies deceiving the patient (Shorter 1985, 245–46). However, the inert sugar pills of yesterday, claims Shorter, have been replaced by powerful drugs used for the same purpose—particularly tranquilizers and antidepressants—to cure by suggestion. When patients take prescribed medications not medically indicated, the placebo effect may still operate, but there will also be organic reactions because the substances ingested are not inert.

Although there is much uncertainty as to exactly how the placebo effect works, the process is culturally relative and its success relies on the patient's socialization, beliefs, and trust in the healer. Berton Roueche, a medical reporter, finds that the placebo receives its power from the "infinite capacity of the human mind for self-deception" (quoted in Cousins 1981 [1979]). As Jamaicans say, belief can cure, and belief can kill.

Daniel Moerman argues that we should refer more accurately to the placebo effect as "the meaning response" (2002). This is because an inactive ("fake") pill cannot, by definition, produce the effect; rather, its meaning does. That is, a person's culturally directed interpretation regarding a pill's color, or name, or shape, or the context of dispensing (or etc.) is what underwrites biomedically inexplicable—but physiologically measureable—healing (or pain reduction, or etc.) in certain situations.

For instance, recent research has shown that knowledge about price can support healing; in a U.S.-based placebo pill pain reduction study, subjects given the placebo but told it was rather expensive ($2.50 per pill) fared even better than subjects given the placebo but told it was only 10¢ (Waber et al. 2008). The cultural adage "you get what you pay for" or the assumption that things that cost more are better may have been at work. Similarly, studies regarding the role of the built environment in facilitating or impeding healing in hospital settings have supported the use of features such as garden views for patient rooms (Ulrich 1984, 2006).We have much to learn about the underlying physiological pathways and mechanisms that placebos can activate. Notwithstanding, if we knew more about the connotations that have helped make placebos so effective in various cultural contexts, including those that support ritual nonbiomedical healing, we could begin to leverage the placebo effect to optimize the meaning response and improve patient outcomes.

The pressure that cultural attitudes and understandings can exert on health cannot be underestimated—as many successful healers know. Therapeutically, the patient must have a role in anything that has to do with his or her health, illness, living, or dying (Zola 1983). A patient's trust in his or her physician may serve as a placebo-like therapeutic mechanism (Shorter 1985); however, under some conditions, and when too much trust is given at the cost of limiting the patients' willingness or ability to accept the responsibility for making choices, it may do more harm than good. The "manipulation of the patient" (238) and abuse of trust, even if thought to be in the patient's best interest, raises important ethical questions.

EMIC AND ETIC POINTS OF VIEW

In classifying personalistic and naturalistic healing approaches, we can refer to the **emic**, or insider's point of view, as contrasted with the **etic**, or scientific outsider's supposedly objective, universalized way of seeing the world. For example, the organic contents of a personalistic medicine can and often do contain compounds that can knock out bacteria or otherwise help in healing. However, the cure is not *seen* from the insider's point of view as hinging on naturalistic action but, rather, on the actions taken to loosen the hold of illness as personalistically acquired. And when this is the case, we must classify the approach as personalistic.

The same rule can be applied in classifying some medicines that are thought to effect organic cures but that outsiders might say work through personalistic action (e.g., through pleasing god or removing spirits from the body, or by the placebo effect). If practitioners and patients attribute the effectiveness of the treatment to naturalistic factors, then naturalistic medicine it is. As outsiders are always positioned in some sociocultural context and so are prone to judge health systems by their own criteria, the best approach is to take the emic point of view as the classificatory key for attaining the best possible understanding of the patient's position—of what patients might be thinking—and doing—about their treatment regimen.

CONTEMPORARY U.S. MEDICINE: THE OUTER FRINGES

Systems of health care, as we have seen, are constantly in flux; they may borrow from other systems and change or evolve with opportunity and necessity. Even in biomedicine, new systems have emerged, for example, in borrowing from the vitalist branch of the equilibrium tradition. **Vitalism** involves a kind of energy or healing force that is activated to reestablish balance and harmony.

Once considered quackery by physicians and nurses, **therapeutic touch** (or hand-mediated energetic healing) is one therapy from a vitalist tradition that has strongly attracted members of the nursing profession. This is perhaps because nurses must typically deal with the whole patient in all degrees of suffering, and for much longer time spans than most doctors do.

Therapeutic touch is based on a belief in a universal healing energy, which is activated through touch, use of the hands, and the focus of the mind. In Western science, the most closely related concepts are physicists' descriptions of quantum and electromagnetic fields, which closely resemble the descriptions of the vitalist systems. Although the therapy looks odd to our culturally conditioned eyes, sometimes involving waving the hands over another person, the results of application have been statistically significant (Slater 1996, 133). Even though much research is needed on outcomes, the technique has produced demonstrable relief for real suffering in patients receiving chemotherapy and those suffering with asthma, migraines, and symptoms associated with HIV (133).

SUFFERING AND QUACKERY'S APPEAL

Physicians confronted with almost any form of therapy not sanctioned by the medical profession or considered "scientifically validated" are quick to cry "quack." But complementary modalities are not ipso facto quackery. Quackery proper is based on false claims of cure and alleviation, promoted as "scientifically based" when this really is not so. The best definition of quackery thus hinges on the *intent* to deceive.

People of all ages, cultures, socioeconomic status, and educational level can be victims. Those who are highly educated, in fact, seem just as prone to fall for promises of pain relief and cure, sexual potency, rejuvenation, unlimited energy, and a slim silhouette. People who are desperately sick and for whom biomedicine has no answers, such as people with incurable cancer, may feel they have nothing to lose in searching out other alternatives. These people form a lucrative clientele for those who purposely exploit hope, misery, and desperation. The industry is booming with products promising cures for everything from arthritis, cancer, and heart disease to diabetes, hypertension, and AIDS.

There is a fine line between protection from the dangers of medical fraud and the open-minded consideration of possible efficacy and the enlistment of complementary therapies in treating the whole person. Socioeconomic conditions within our society are also creating pressure for a reevaluation of complementary modalities as both cost effective and efficacious when combined with biomedicine.

Education and even legislation have failed to curtail medical fraud because they do not touch the root of the problem. People are not only multicultural, they are multidimensional; as long as biomedicine ministers to only one of those dimensions, people will search for additional or alternative means for fulfilling human needs. A truly complementary approach, one that blends biomedical and alternative modalities, would minister to all the aspects of human suffering; then, perhaps, quackery would lose much of its appeal.

Albert Schweitzer, after years of medical experience in Africa, observed that "the [indigenous healer] succeeds for the same reason all the rest of us succeed. Each patient carries his own doctor inside him. They come to us not knowing that truth. We are at our best when we give the doctor who resides within each patient a chance to go to work" (quoted in Cousins 1981 [1979], 69).

We may all carry that "doctor inside," but when really ill, we also must often seek help from those with further knowledge and expertise to help. In the next chapter, we will explore the currently dominant medical system and how cultural elements were vital in its development. We will also examine how biomedicine is very much a part of culture, as well as a culture in itself.

FOR DISCUSSION

1. Describe the social structure of health care practice in the United States with reference to its various sectors and the different types of health care workers that occupy them. What value does this exercise have for illuminating how health care functions (or does not)? Why might it (or why might it not) be a good idea to think of health care workers as occupying different social positions or sectors?

2. In what way does Galenic medicine survive in the current construction of biomedicine? List some examples of humoral-style views and practices that you have observed in biomedical settings. How are these different from (or similar to) humoral-style ideas

and practices carried out in your home in the name of good health?

3. All health practitioners should fit into the two main groups and the nine subgroups offered in this chapter (five subgroups are naturalistic; four are personalistic). What criteria would you use to categorize a practitioner as belonging to one or the other main group? What criteria would you use to categorize her or him within that grouping? Make a list of practitioners that you have patronized and try to class them accordingly. What function does classification serve?

4. What are some of the reasons that people have for visiting differing types of practitioners? What factors make them turn away from others? Discuss quackery and how, as a label, it affects the use and acceptance of various therapies.

CHAPTER 5

Biomedicine: Emergence and Evolution in Cultural Context

GOAL: Examine the development of the American medical system, including its multicultural roots and related contributions, from an ethnohistorical perspective.

GOAL: Understand the difference between the scientific paradigm and medical care per se, and describe the ways in which they both are both cultural constructions.

GOAL: Identify various cultural issues related to biomedicine, including its achievements and limitations; become familiar with related evolving arguments and models.

A series of events culminating in the Flexner report of 1910 resulted in establishing allopathic [biomedical] professional knowledge as the dominant form—a transformation that quickly delegitimized all other kinds of knowledge, putting the newly defined medical profession in a position of cultural authority, economic power, and political influence.... The power of authoritative knowledge is not that it is correct but that it counts.

(Jordan 1993, 153–54, emphasis in original)

Science is generally taken for granted in the United States as the ultimate authority regarding what is true and what is not. Science entails using the

scientific method of investigation, which consists of observing, hypothesizing, and testing expected relationships and predicting outcomes, then revising expectations when discrepancies arise. Science is typified by reliance on **experimental** methods, the goals of which are to test hypotheses about the relationship(s) between two or more **variables** (discrete influences or states). The dominant system of medicine in the United States, biomedicine, is based upon this scientific paradigm.

But the scientific **paradigm** (a set of guiding theories and methods) is only one means of understanding the world, and giving it primacy could be considered ethnocentric. Consider, for example, the Zen Buddhist, who considers all aspects of the observable and unobservable world as an integrated whole and rejects the idea that such a method of breaking things down into parts and studying their relationships can help to control or understand the world (Johnson 1996, 3).

Still, science, as practiced through the scientific method, has allowed us to make great discoveries and to gain insights into and understanding of countless phenomena and has resulted in innumerable products and technologies that would have been impossible without it. It is precisely this argument that supports, and in fact requires, the promotion of scientific literacy in the educational system.

However, like all cultural systems, the medical system is a human invention, linked to all other aspects of our sociocultural context. Science is only one element in medicine's development and character. This chapter explores the processes of medicine's evolution and change in relation to the sociocultural context.

THE MULTICULTURAL BACKGROUND

The United States was colonized by a great diversity of peoples. New arrivals faced the common problems of illness and disease, but brought with them their own perceptions and approaches to health, illness, and treatment. The modern American medical system thus derived from a multiculturally based diversity of folk traditions and practices and evolved into a dominative system based on the **biomedical model** (grounded in the scientific method). This model duplicates American class, racial/ethnic, and gender relations, and constitutes the standard by which all other medical systems are measured (Baer 1989, 1110).

The alternative folk-based or sectarian systems that did not fit this model were eventually excluded from the system. Only those philosophies and therapies validated by the scientific method and sanctioned by mainstream or orthodox medicine would be seen to have value in healing. American medical pluralism, however, persists in the diversity of health care systems. As Baer (2001) notes, "Biomedicine's dominance over rival medical systems has never been absolute. The state, which primarily serves the interests of the corporate class, must periodically make concessions to subordinate social groups in the interests of maintaining social order and the capitalist mode of production" (43). Whether and which of these systems remain on the fringe, disappear, become co-opted by the dominant system, or become integrated into a more inclusive system remains to be seen.

HISTORY, CULTURE, AND THE HEALTH CARE SYSTEM

History shows that numerous factors and events, evolving within a multicultural framework around a core of institutionalized patterns of values and beliefs, have influenced the direction and construction of the American health care system. Prior to the late nineteenth and early twentieth centuries, however, medical histories were not critical histories, but were written from a medical point of view and were read basically by doctors for information on how to treat patients (Sigerist 1960 [1947]). By 1929, when medicine was becoming more "scientific," the histories began to focus on the concerns of medical humanists, of how to maintain patient-centered traditions in the face of scientific objectivism—concerns still with us today.

Within the last few decades, the questions addressed by medical historiography have begun to concern the role and nature of medicine within culture. Medical knowledge has come to include social history, involving relations with patients, moral systems, and social responses to disease as well as knowledge of disease itself. In addition, "the study of epidemic disease entailed an inquiry into how episodic and extraordinary medical events reflected and produced changes in the organization of cultural norms and values, institutions and intellect" (Brandt 1991, 202).

But medical history has often been constructed around the impressive and progressive accomplishments of science as a history of triumph over ignorance and suffering. Without question, the astounding progress of biomedical science has made life longer and better for many. However, the emerging ethnohistorical framework, with its emphasis on social factors, gives us another view—one that helps to explain this progress at a more human level, and to illuminate the myriad of problems that have accompanied it.

It has been widely shown that social forces shape or construct our perceptions and experiences of health, illness, and healing, a process known generally as **social constructionism** (Lupton 1994). There are numerous definitions of social constructionism within sociology and anthropology; however, we support the notion of a contextual construction, which recognizes biological realities, but stresses the social context. This approach considers the influences of both human interaction and political-economic factors on development and meaning of health, illness, and care, which also must include the traditional roots of the system (for an extended discussion of social constructionism and this approach, see Brown 1995).

ROOTS OF THE U.S. HEALTH CARE SYSTEM

The term "ethnomedicine" or, more plainly and commonly, "folk medicine" often is used by lay people (or health workers unschooled regarding cultural issues) to designate health-related beliefs and practices of traditional societies. **Folk medicine** thus might be defined by its contrast to modern, scientific medicine—the official medicine of the industrialized world. It is from folk, or "unofficial" medicine, however, that many patients derive their attitudes, values, and decisions about medical care in general (Hufford 1992, 14). The United States has been a multicultural nation from the beginning, and "all medical traditions in the pluralistic cultural environment of the United States affect one another deeply and constantly" (Hufford 1994, 117).

The stereotype of folk medicine as isolated from the mainstream is therefore not at all correct. Folk and official medicines even share certain metaphors. Both may view certain diseases as malevolent invaders that "attack" the body, which then mounts a defense to "fight off" or "drive out" the invaders (Magner 1992, 12). Folk traditions represent "a universal set of efforts to cope with illness in ways that go beyond—but do not necessarily conflict with—what modern medicine has to offer" (Hufford 1992, 15).

Another example of the similarities of folk and biomedical healing is in the use of symbols. Symbolic healing was and is a part of folk practice and can be seen as operant in all healing through a type of "universal" or deeper structure at the psychological level, which utilizes "culturally specific symbol imagery" (Dow 1986). Religious healing, magical healing, and Western psychotherapy all incorporate versions of this common structure, regardless of culture. Dow explains that "symbolic healing becomes possible when a particularized mythic world exists [or is established] for both the therapist [healer] and the patient and when the patient accepts the power of the therapist to define the patient's relation to that world. The therapist [shaman, healer, psychotherapist] then attaches the patient's emotions to transactional symbols and manipulates these symbols [to effect healing]" (1986, 66).

Overlap of folk with biomedicine may also occur through diffusion or appropriation. **Medical syncretism** is the process of blending another group's medical remedies, knowledge, and techniques of treatment and diagnosis of illness with one's own. Syncretism occurred, for example, when access to various European healing methods and remedies familiar to colonists in the New World were limited or nonexistent, and new diseases were encountered. Indigenous knowledge and therapies then became extremely important to the colonizers.

Native Americans, generally quite healthy before new diseases were introduced by Europeans (Kunitz 1983), had wide knowledge of the ailments and remedies indigenous to their own environments. Twaddle and Hessler (1987) note that "the Native American healer frequently assumed the superordinate role of teacher and doctor to whites, an almost quixotic notion according to modern conceptions that define Native American healing as primitive and folksy" (177). Others took the view of one highly biased medical historian, U.S. Army Colonel P. M. Ashburn, that "the savage Indians and the Negroes contributed little or nothing of value to any branch of medicine, and from them we received a mass of superstition and ignorance that reinforced and strengthened what we had brought from Europe, a heritage that still plagues us" (quoted in Vogel 1990, 6).

Although general Native American healing philosophies differ from white Western biomedical views of health and illness, there is considerable variation across indigenous groups. Native American acquaintance with the physiological effects of a large number of drugs was extensive and formed the groundwork for the development of such modern medications as anesthetics, insulin, antibiotics, and even birth control pills (Vogel 1990). That knowledge—as well as techniques such as sweat baths, surgery, poultices, and mineral soaks—form an important legacy for American biomedical practice. Divergent philosophies and a Western ethnocentric orientation have blinded us to this heritage, causing us to lose "some of the ability to assess where we have been and where our medical care system is taking us" (Twaddle and Hessler 1987, 177).

When we do acknowledge the past, we typically do so with generic examples relating to Native American, European, African American, Asian, and Hispanic folk medicine. But these ethnic designations each refer to a wide variety of cultures, each with its own approach to health, illness, and medical care. Syncretism occurred among them, as well as between them and other populations with whom they had cultural contact. There was also an ongoing adaptation to new geographical environments and resources for all immigrant cultures, as well as a complex and intricate relationship with social institutions, culture, and social structure.

FOLK CONTRIBUTIONS

There were many reasons for the preservation, adaptation and use of diverse folk remedies in America during colonial times. First, very few physicians trained in European medical schools were available in the seventeenth-century colonies. In addition, colonial society was steeped in democratic and egalitarian ideals. The democratic, antielitist attitudes of the times supported the notion that the practice of medicine was a matter of common sense, to which all had access. Health care was generally provided within social networks, came out of oral traditions passed down through families and friends, and was not seen as the property of an elite few who charged for their services. The family was the source of care, and women the main caregivers.

Rural isolation also necessitated self-sufficiency: Households generally provided for all their own needs, including food, shelter, clothing, and health care. In any case, many people simply could not afford medical care from a physician. Because many people lived in isolated rural areas, paying for care included transportation costs that often amounted to more than the doctor's fee. In addition, considering the level of professional medical knowledge, doctors could generally offer little that people could not provide for themselves.

Another reason for turning to folk-based care was that up until the late 1800s and the advent of a more scientifically based and predictably beneficial medicine, seeking professional medical care involved a highly calculated risk, because, even though several states eventually passed perfunctory licensing laws, "in 1846 almost any man with an elementary education could take a course of lectures for one or two winters, pass an examination and thereby automatically achieve the right to practice medicine by state law" (Shryock 1966 [1947], 152). Thus due to patient experience and doctors' reputations, few people had much faith in physicians' abilities. Even officially trained physicians could not always agree as to the proper methods and courses of treatment (as is still often the case today).

Folk medicine and self-care were most practical and quite simply necessary. When people did require additional care, however, there was a variety of theories, treatments, and practitioners from which they could choose.

THE SECTARIANS

Various philosophies and approaches to medical care originating both at home and abroad were popular during the nineteenth century. Some were labeled **sects** due to their exclusionary nature, dogmatic attitudes, and the intense loyalty of their followers. The sects each claimed to have discovered the true nature of disease and illness and the proper approach to curing and healing. They may have arisen partly as a response to what were considered "heroic cures" and therapies of orthodox physicians, which included such unpleasant and potentially dangerous practices as bleeding, purging, vomiting, sweating, blistering, and liberal use of such mineral compounds as calomel (mild mercurous chloride), later found to be highly toxic (Sullivan 1994).

Primary among these early sectarian groups were the Thomsonians, the eclectics who were basically botanic doctors, and homeopaths. Osteopathy, Christian Science, faith healing, and chiropractic appeared around the turn of the century and into the 1900s, as new sects replaced old (for an extended discussion of these medical sects, see Micozzi 1996b).

Abraham Flexner (1910), in his classic assessment of the status of American medical education (to be discussed later), saw sects as an inevitable and even logical opposition to preconceived notions (other than their own) about causes and treatments for illness. Orthodox medical philosophy and practice, sometimes termed **allopathic** medicine because of its focus on symptom alleviation, was, at the time, just as sectarian as the rest (Starr 1982). Flexner felt that with the establishment of a scientific basis for diagnosis and treatment, all philosophies would be submitted to rigorous scientific examination. He predicted that the sectarian approaches would either die out (their schools in the United States were already reduced, and enrollment was declining) or be co-opted into the modern medical fold. His predictions were to prove only partially correct (see Starr 1982).

THE ORTHODOX PROFESSION OF MEDICINE

In colonial times, doctors (those trained in or possessing some official medical knowledge, who identified themselves as physicians), especially those trained in Europe, viewed the practice of medicine as a basis for social status and aristocratic privilege rather than a profession to serve those in need. The title "physician" thus entailed aristocratic patronage from the wealthy and powerful and legal protection as practitioners—benefits and privileges that were simply not available to doctors in a democratically inclined American colonial society where equality was the ideal.

Doctors in America therefore found themselves in competition with lay practitioners, folk medicine, and eventually other (sectarian) systems of therapy. Doctors also competed with **patent medicine** companies, which sold their trademarked medical preparations directly to the public, offering their own explanations of causes and easy cures for a multitude of ailments from arthritis to baldness.

Competition was augmented by the fact that the demand for physicians was essentially low at the same time that physicians, due to the lax restrictions on entry into the field of medicine and low cost of a degree, were in oversupply. By 1846, due to strong competition, "the excess of physicians was such that many young graduates failed to secure a decent practice and abandoned the profession" (Shryock 1966, 156).

Some doctors declared that medical discoveries should be disseminated to the lay public in easily understood language, thereby providing the lay public with greater self-healing knowledge. Other doctors, however, saw medicine as a privileged profession, with specialized knowledge that conferred status and should not be shared with those who could not understand its complexities. This position reflects an early attempt to use **authoritative knowledge**—knowledge that "builds and reflects power relationships" to construct a stronger professional base and what Jordan calls a "community of practice" (1993, 153). Drawing on the work of various social theorists, Jordan relates this move toward autonomy to a cross-culturally identified process,

> whereby the authority of [a] particular knowledge system and the power relations supporting it and benefitting from it come to be perceived not as socially constructed, relative, and often coercive,

but as natural, legitimate, and in the best interest of all parties. This process makes the achieved order of the world appear to be a fact of nature, with the consequence that the dominant positions in that order are also a fact of nature, and hence cannot be changed.

(Jordan 1993, 153)

While physicians established a position of status and privilege through professional identity and licensure, science was to provide a more solid foundation. It was to open the way to a "legitimate" complexity, moving medicine out of the realm of lay understanding and common sense and, ultimately, to complete professional autonomy.

Science, however, was only one link in the chain of events. Starr (1982) links the development of the modern medical system with the rise and increasing dominance of the medical profession in the United States and notes that dominance was actually achieved before science had contributed much to the doctors' capabilities for addressing disease. Early scientific discoveries were important, but made little impact on actual medical care. Practicing physicians had little to offer their patients until the catalyst of World War II.

The impotence of medicine before World War II was sensed by many. One physician, who could envision enormous possibilities, described the time as "an era of very little light" and remarked upon the need to sit down with the patient and listen—"to comfort and console always" (J. Dunbar Shields, quoted in Kaufman 1993, 151)—because in most cases, doctors could do little else. Another, describing his practice between 1936 and 1942, observed, "For cases of infection, there were no antibiotics when I first started in practice. I would try to support the patient's nutrition and morale and physical cleanliness. ... Almost all organic diseases of the nervous system were untreatable" (Saul Jarcho, quoted in Kaufman 1993, 161). This emphasizes the importance of nonbiomedical factors in biomedicine's achievement of dominance.

GROWTH OF THE SCIENTIFIC MEDICAL MODEL

A number of significant discoveries and events are generally cited as instrumental in establishing the centrality and dominance of scientific medicine, which consequently discredited other systems of healing. Louis Pasteur's germ theory of disease, the founding of the American Medical Association, Abraham Flexner's report on the state of American medical education, and the development of the hospital system, plus later rapid growth of technology after World War II had major cultural impacts upon treatment modalities and the context and delivery of health care in the United States.

THE GERM THEORY

In the 1860s and 1870s, Louis Pasteur, a French chemist, isolated the organisms responsible for major infectious diseases, including deadly rabies. His formulation of the germ theory had a tremendous impact upon a broad range of scientific medical research and development (Magner 1992).

The **germ theory**, initially embraced as *the* primary explanation for the spread of disease, was powerful, appealing, and simplistic. Once accepted, the theory generated a great deal of enthusiasm and stimulated the search for disease-causing germs. But the idea that germs are monocausal agents (one germ for each disease) proved to be in error. For a time, the blind acceptance of this idea kept researchers from exploring other avenues of causation, such as additional pathological, social, cultural, and environmental factors that turned out to be vital to understanding and controlling the disease process. At this time, patients' cultural backgrounds, beliefs, values, and traditions were considered inconsequential to diagnosis and treatment.

The germ theory achieved great advances; it changed causal attribution and related practices and added to knowledge about the sources of contagion and the health-and-illness connections between and among communities and even nations. Diseases could now be scientifically classified according to perceived causes rather than only signs and symptoms, and illness was no longer explained only by physical or social conditions or as a divine punishment for moral infractions. After the germ theory, however, "the culture of the organism, not of the patient, was the important determinant of sickness (Kunitz 1994, 176).

THE AMERICAN MEDICAL ASSOCIATION

Even before the discovery of germs, physicians pursued their quest for control and professionalization of medicine. They established medical societies in some states during the first half of the nineteenth century, and in 1847, they met in Philadelphia to establish the American Medical Association (AMA). This was a key step in the professionalization process.

A reorganization of the AMA in 1902 established branch societies on the local, state, and territorial levels. Local societies had the arbitrary discretion to expel or deny membership to any physician, and thus could determine membership qualifications and enforce conformity. This enabled the profession to monitor and control a widely dispersed membership.

Having a professional association allowed physicians to better organize their attack on competitive elements, as well as to further develop the scientific basis for medicine and the legitimacy of the scientific approach. They still disagreed with and battled each other on all sorts of medical, philosophical, and organizational issues, but the AMA provided a forum where interests could be discussed and defended, and also served as a potential pressure group for future political and policy endeavors.

Still, newspaper headlines and articles of the mid-1800s provide evidence that the early status of the medical profession was not at all high. For instance, the editor of the *Cincinnati Medical Observer* of 1857 was quoted as pointing out that many "speak of the Medical Profession as a body of jealous, quarrelsome men, whose chief delight is in the annoyance and ridicule of each other" (quoted in Shryock 1966, 151). It was not until near the beginning of the twentieth century that the status of members of the American medical profession really began to improve. Its potential power by that time, however, was considerable.

The power of the AMA was used to raise and maintain academic and scientific standards, but it was also used to consolidate power and further its own interests, including the economic position of the medical profession. It also helped to secure the autonomous right to define and enforce the restraints, as well as the standards of practice, with a freedom known to very few professions. Thus, there emerged what Freidson called "a new tyranny which sincerely expresses itself in the language of humanitarianism and which imposes its own values on others for what it sees to be their own good" (1970, 382).

Another event supporting professional dominance occurred in 1910 with the publication of the Flexner Report. A broader view of that event reveals not only its role in the establishment of scientific medicine and standardized medical education, but its links with social-structural elements and capitalist cultural values as well.

THE FLEXNER REPORT

In 1908, the AMA contracted with the Carnegie Foundation for a study of American medical education to be conducted by Abraham

Flexner, an administrator and educator. The goal of the study was to standardize and raise the status of American medical education. Because the cost of a scientific medical education was beyond most students, and capital investment and operating costs for schools were beyond the means of the profession, it was recognized that the money would have to come from the rich. Both philanthropists and the public would therefore have to be convinced that modern medicine was a field worthy of their support.

Professional medical reformers were well aware of the need for a strategy consistent with current historical forces. This meant offering investment opportunities in conquering disease and the promise of international status and leadership to investors (E. Brown 1979, 141). In keeping with the new scientific discoveries and inventions in the industrial sector, which promised growth and profits, the time had come to promote "scientific medicine."

The resulting **Flexner Report** of 1910 marked a historical turning point in medical education. The movement for medical school reform had actually begun in 1870 at Harvard. The AMA's Council on Medical Education had even done a preliminary survey in 1907, which served as the basis for Flexner's report, and state medical boards had already begun to upgrade medical school programs (Brown 1979). The report did force the closure of numerous medical schools judged to be of inferior quality, although, due to previous competition and the push for reform, as many schools had closed before as after the report was issued. Unfortunately many of those schools closed had trained women and other minorities.

Before 1910, medical education was open to women in the United States and Canada practically on the same terms as to men. Any woman who desired a medical education should have no difficulty in finding a school, asserted Flexner (1910). With fewer schools and increased competition, however, a growing male hostility within the profession led to policies of women's exclusion. In the matter of medical education, now required for licensure and credentials, "administrators justified outright discrimination against qualified women candidates on the grounds that they would not continue to practice after marriage" (Starr 1982, 124). Medical schools for the next half century after 1910 maintained quotas limiting women to about 5 percent of admissions (124).

A product of a racist society, Flexner supported the medical training of black people, but only in order to care for other blacks—not because they themselves needed care, but because they also came into contact with whites. He emphasized their educational need to concentrate on hygiene rather than surgery. He recommended that out of seven schools for blacks, two schools, Meharry and Howard, be supported and upgraded and the others eliminated. The reduction in black schools resulted in decreased care for black people. In 1910, there was 1 black physician for every 2,883 black people in the United States; by 1942 the ratio was 1 black physician for every 3,377 black people (Brown 1979, 154).

The Flexner Report had positive consequences in educating the public to the benefits of scientific medicine and medical training by standardizing medical education and eliminating the medical diploma mills, which in turn reduced the risk of unproven, incompetent, or fraudulent treatment. However, the report also allowed the medical profession to more closely guard its gates against all but the elite few allowed to become physicians.

With the establishment of uniformity in medical training for all students, and with more uniformity in students themselves (the licensed, medical workforce consisted mostly of white, upper-middle-class males), the profession became more homogeneous. Higher costs of a medical education, plus the extended time necessary for study and certification, limited the entry of lower and working classes. Places in medical schools became scarce, and competition for them resulted in policies of discrimination against Jews, blacks, women, and immigrants. Exclusion from the mainstream meant that alternative philosophies and ideas of diagnosis and treatment could be effectively controlled or suppressed, or could be consigned to a lower class or ethnically identified population. The exclusionary race-class-sex composition of the profession persisted until the opening up of medical education with affirmative action programs in the 1960s and 1970s, and had profound consequences for the development of the health care system in the United States.

THE FLEXNER LEGACY

Taking into account the larger context and social dynamics of the time, the Flexner Report can be seen as an attempt by the AMA to "attain and maintain ideological hegemony over the other sects of medicine that were still extant at the time"; it also helped to "solidify the alliance between the capitalist class and the AMA and to establish the dominance of the researcher over the practitioner" (Berliner 1975, 589). Further, the report established a new medical paradigm—that of the body as machine with an emphasis on research, therapy, and repair (pathology and cure). "That this conception," notes

Berliner, "is a reflection of the larger economic system is not to be considered an accident" (590).

Berliner's conclusion (as well as the similar conclusions of others, e.g., Martin, 1987; Zola 1983; Baer 1989) is based on the presence of vested capitalist interests in legitimating the existing social structure of the times, with its emphasis on scientism, and the subordination of means of production, including medical care institutions, to capital accumulation. Implementation of the Flexner Report was undertaken by the nine largest philanthropic organizations in the United States, which together gave more than $150 million to particular medical schools over the 20 years following the emergence of the report (Berliner 1975, 590).

In the pre-World War II era, philanthropic foundations contributed to strengthening medical schools, biomedical research, and public health programs. In 1940, foundation grants totaled $12 million, or 30 percent of the total national expenditures in this area. In the postwar era, however, philanthropic donations were far outstripped by funding from private insurance, federal, state, and local governments, and consumer out-of-pocket payments. Thus it can be argued that the foundations have not been the "movers and shakers" they were thought to be (Ginzberg 1990). Still, the early alliance of medicine with wealthy capitalist interests profoundly affected the development of the system: Large investments are not made with no hope of return. Many within the AMA recognized the dangers of alliances with strong capitalist interests who would then have a say in designating areas of priorities in education and research (Brown 1979). These areas could be chosen to provide investment opportunities with bigger payoffs and to support the class structure rather than according to need. As Berliner suggests, "The problems that plague the field of medicine today no doubt emerge dialectically from the attempt made in 1910 to shore up a medical system also beset with contradictions and conflicts" (1975, 590).

As the system continues to evolve, it must be noted that the power and influence of the AMA is not unilateral. Medicare in the 1960s, for example, was opposed by the AMA and yet became law. The AMA was also excluded from participation in the Clinton health reform planning and was treated as another "special interest group." The organizational resources of expertise, financing, and structure enable the AMA to play a role in offering policy recommendations and guidance to physicians, although with increasing numbers of players and policy issues, that role has dwindled (Hafferty and Light 1995,

138; see also Cockerham 2010). Mainstream medicine, nevertheless, still dominates the health care system.

THE DEVELOPMENT OF THE HOSPITAL SYSTEM

The growth and dominance of mainstream medicine also was fueled by hospitals. They provided a laboratory for the science of medicine and for the physician's practice, creating an institution that would become central to the medical care delivery system.

Before 1850, hospitals served the indigent poor and acute cases or short-stay patients, while chronic cases, the incurable, the insane, and those with communicable diseases were sent to public institutions. These people were not considered appropriate subjects for hospital admissions, and would take up spaces that might better be used by those who could be cured or benefit from treatment (Rosen 1974).

In the mid-nineteenth century, various religious or ethnic institutions were developed for specific diseases such as tuberculosis, for categories of the population such as women and children, and for various medical sects such as homeopathy. These specialty hospitals served several purposes: They offered internships and residencies for minority physicians who were denied entry elsewhere, and allowed them a facility for attending their patients. Specialty hospitals also eased the fears of various religious and ethnic minorities that cultural customs, beliefs, and rituals—such as last rites, confession, or Kosher diet requirements—would not be honored or would be ridiculed in other hospitals.

Cultural separatism offered at least some opportunity for educational advancement and sensitive, culturally relative care for minority populations, but at a price: It did nothing to change the discriminatory structure of society and social institutions or to lessen the intolerance and insensitivity of health care providers toward other cultural groups. Separatism thus served a stabilizing function by not upsetting the socially dominant, very "unscientific" racist and ethnocentric structure (see Krause 1977).

The development of the American hospital system was basically unplanned, with no conscious efforts at coordination, but it did reflect a definite pattern of class relations (Starr 1982). This was especially true in the elite private hospitals where staff were strictly controlled, and patients were either very poor (for teaching purposes) or very rich (for revenue). The centralization of both learning and practice within a hospital setting made it much easier to maintain a particular standard of medical education with control of curriculum, training, and require-ments. The role of the hospital, however, evolved quite drastically with the advent of World War II.

WORLD WAR II: A TURNING POINT

By the 1940s, biomedicine's dominance was more or less secured. However, the war made scientific medicine a national asset and an institution, and served as a catalyst for a boom in scientific research that would further define the culture of mainstream medicine. Research produced medical discoveries that lowered the military death rate and could be transferred to the populace. The United States emerged from the war as a formidable economic and military power. Scientific medicine became associated with victory, the conquest of infectious diseases, prosperity, and leadership of the free world—biomedicine was American.

The 1940s and 1950s were a golden age for antibiotics. The physicians' arsenal for combating disease was filled to overflowing with new miracle drugs, and the military metaphors used in descrip-tions of medical victories over disease fit nicely with the victories of World War II. Penicillin, whose development was closely associated with military needs and objectives, proved to be effective against venereal diseases as well as battle injuries, and streptomycin was found to be effective against tuberculosis. These advances fueled the search for new drugs and their potential profits.

The new, scientifically tested medications were impressively effective, but diverted attention from and further discredited folk remedies and traditional forms of medical care. Use of the new drugs became a status symbol, while folk practices became associated with ignorance and superstition. Biomedicine developed a heavy reliance upon the new drug therapies for treatment and cure, despite early (and presciently accurate) warnings that overuse and misuse could produce dangerous side effects and drug-resistant organisms (see Garrett 1994). The use of scientifically developed and approved drugs as a major medical therapy, however, was firmly established.

With a high number of wounded military personnel returning to the United States, patients could no longer be warehoused in nontreat-ment facilities. Moreover, the growing arsenal of drugs and treatments increased biomedicine's potential for cures and rehabilitations. In turn, hospitals moved from being religious centers that served the poor and offered a place to die to being centers for physician practice and advanced medical technology, serving all members of society. They no longer discriminated openly according to race and ethnicity, or wealth and poverty, although some specialty designations persisted, including women's hospitals, children's hospitals, and psychiatric hospitals. Further, the poor were generally relegated to the public voluntary, nonprofit or government-owned hospitals, while paying patients were more likely to be sent to private, for-profit hospitals.

The field of psychiatry also emerged from the war with newfound status, and social problems and conditions began to be defined in medical terms. Various categories previously not considered by most as medical, such as depression, began to be viewed as medical problems to be treated. This viewpoint was supported by an alliance of liberalism, which was focused on promoting the public good, and biomedicine, which broadened the need for medical research, hospital construction, and other forms of resource development (Starr 1982).

With postwar economic growth and prosperity, the advance of scientific medicine promised health and well-being through its own progress without any need for a restructuring of society. Government supported its programs, but refrained from any intervention in policy. Physicians were seen as "professionals," requiring autonomy (cf. Turner 1995), which was consistent with prevailing cultural and political beliefs.

The public service orientation of biomedicine, its ethical basis, and claim of specialized knowledge justified nonintervention (no regulation) by government. The Marxist interpretation that professional groups (including medical ones) under state protection actually support the capitalist enterprise by legitimizing conditions of production (including health-related ones) through monitoring and maintaining surveillance of the working class (Turner 1995, 130; also see Foucault 1975 [1963]) would also justify nonintervention by the state. The emerging structure of the United States' dominant medical system thus remained intact.

THE ROAD TO ALTERNATIVES

The belief in growth without conflict continued until the 1960s, when flaws in the biomedical system began to become too apparent. The goal of biomedicine was challenged as people who recognized the benefits and need for medical care could not afford it. The system responded to needs in an ad hoc fashion.

The biomedical system that had evolved by the 1970s was still loosely aligned and basically uncoordinated. Never designed to serve the poor, it was professionally dominated, scientifically based, cure oriented, and hospital centered, with an open, unregulated fee structure. It was also "overly specialized, overbuilt and overbedded, and insufficiently attentive to the needs of the poor in inner-city and rural areas" (Starr 1982, 382). Health care facilities were unevenly distributed, with resulting inequity in services provided. Physicians tended to opt for practice in wealthier urban areas where large hospitals offered high-tech educational facilities and opportunities, interaction with colleagues, and higher incomes. This resulted in duplication of services in some areas, with few or no services in others.

A two-tier system of care had been created, placing a strain on public hospitals with the poor and indigent, and raising issues of ethics and inequitable quality of care. Many rural and inner-city areas had virtually no access to health care at all. A growing shortage of **primary care physicians** (general practitioners), which resulted from increasing medical specialization, also limited access to family doctors who knew their patients and could coordinate their care.

Three independent national surveys, supported by the Robert Wood Johnson Foundation in 1976, 1982, and 1986, examined the extent of difficulties for individuals seeking medical care. It was found that from 1982 to 1986, even though health status for both blacks and Hispanics was poorer than for whites, these groups were significantly less likely to be hospitalized. In addition, "an estimated one million individuals actually tried to obtain care but did not receive it. The majority of Americans experiencing these difficulties were the poor, uninsured, or minorities" (Freeman et al. 1990, 316). The emerging value of health care as a "right" carried no accompanying responsibilities for providing it, and people were increasingly taking note.

THE CORPORATE INCURSION AND CONSUMER ACTIVISM

Perhaps the greatest challenge to biomedical professional dominance has come from within the very nature of the capitalist system itself. The history of the growth of corporate (for-profit) medicine, too long and complex to include here, raises the question of whether medicine with the primary emphasis on profit is or can be consistent with the service orientation of medicine as it relates to the good of humanity and the alleviation of suffering.

By the 1960s and 1970s, biomedicine had the potential of a growth industry, but with increasing costs and poor management it was floundering. The 1980s and 1990s saw attempts to restructure the system with the entry of corporate managed care, including health maintenance organizations, group practice, preferred provider organizations, case managers, and other means to hold down costs. As health care was perceived as profitable, large corporate entities moved into the field to compete with nonprofit entities and expanded into affiliated businesses and industries including hospitals, nursing homes, insurance, hospital equipment, psychiatric services, home health care, and other related areas. This corporate model resulted in managing the system as a business, and health care as a commodity (Starr 1982).

Corporate entry brought with it much needed capital investment and management techniques for securing a profit (Wohl 1984). The view of biomedicine as a profit-making enterprise, however, has further distanced it from a service orientation—and from providing care for those who cannot pay. Doctors find themselves at odds not only with their own patients, but with corporate entities that demand a monetary return on their investments. Professional autonomy becomes co-opted and weakened as doctors find themselves captives of the corporate bottom line (Waitzkin 2000).

Costs were initially reduced. However, consumer dissatisfaction and physician objections, as well as follow-on cost increases, have weakened the managed care model, resulting in less control, more consumer-physician choice, and more rising costs (Mechanic 2004).

For their part, with access to medical care a growing concern, consumers have become disaffected with the biomedical profession and still-rising prices. The resultant explosion of consumer-directed information, as seen in the wide availability of books, newsletters, television programs, magazine articles, public classes, and now Internet resources, is educating the population with regard to prevention and care. The early settlers' self-help ideal has reappeared—not so much as common sense, but as personal interest in education and knowledge aimed at health maintenance and illness prevention and a desire to gain more control in decision making and more value for the medical dollar (Keckley and Eselius 2009; Salmon 1984). A growing portion of consumers searching for value even are electing to travel to other countries for their care (Keckley and Underwood 2008; Sobo 2009b).

As noted in Chapter 4, consumers have also rediscovered and are showing great interest in what are considered **complementary** or **alternative** medicine (**CAM**) systems or forms of care. They may be used instead of, but are more generally used in conjunction with, mainstream therapies. Many of these additional systems of health care have simply coexisted with biomedicine like islands in the medical mainstream. Herbs, massage, chiropractic, acupuncture, homeopathy, faith healing, and other therapies offer alternatives when biomedical care is unaffordable, unobtainable, or unsatisfactory, and may be complementary when used with other therapies. Some CAM options thrive primarily within subcultural groupings of poor racial and ethnic minorities, but are by no means limited to them (Cockerham 2010). Today, about 4 in 10 Americans use CAM (Barnes, Bloom, and Nahin 2008), although most do not tell their doctors (Eisenberg et al. 1993; see also Prussing et al. 2004).

However, this does not necessarily mean the beginning of a more medically pluralistic system: "As long as the corporate class and its state sponsors dictate health policy, the American medical system will remain a dominative one and continue to reflect social relations in the larger society" (Baer 1989, 1111). Baer also notes, in relation to incorporation of CAM systems with the biomedical system, that "an emancipatory 'therapeutic alliance' would require an egalitarian relationship between representatives of different medical systems, one that would transcend the hierarchical structure of the American dominative medical system" (2001, 188).

Instead, many social forces are at work in favor of incorporating CAM into the mainstream healing system. Goldstein (2000) suggests that as health care becomes commodified, dissatisfaction with biomedicine, high costs, and media support will all function to integrate CAM therapies into the mainstream. Various CAM modalities are also being tested, researched, and evaluated through the federal government's National Center for Complementary and Alternative Medicine. As Goldstein notes, "To the extent that alternative medicine can turn pathology into opportunity, it will continue to gain acceptance in society" (295).

As for the future of acceptance, use, and integration of CAM, Goldstein proposes that corporate control of media and managed care "is one of the driving forces behind its growing acceptability to the population at large" (2000, 294). CAM is becoming integrated because the same standards that apply to conventional medicine apply to it—cost saving, the generation of economic surpluses, and high profitability.

The gaps and shortcomings of the biomedical model, as well as the need for patient involvement in care (including in in self-care), and the increase in chronic illness have also encouraged a change of attitude within biomedicine. It is therefore necessary to understand biomedicine as a part of culture, and as a culture in itself, as well as to understand its relationship to cultural needs and perceptions.

BIOMEDICINE IN CULTURE

CONSTRUCTING DISEASE, ILLNESS, AND MEDICINE

Almost no one doubts that there is a biological reality. When the normal structure or functioning of the body is disrupted by a disease condition, such as a malignant tumor, it is certainly "there." It can be seen (as through imaging or surgery) and felt (as in symptoms and pain), and it can cause the death of the organism it inhabits or affects. A broken bone is broken; arteries can be plugged; and variations in blood pressure and body temperature can be measured.

Disease conditions can be medically interpreted and treated in numerous ways with some predictability of outcome; some conditions can be cured, some controlled, and others alleviated or made bearable. To an individual, however, a broken bone or a tumor means far more than a simple pathology. A subjective person, not an objective organism, suffers.

Sociologist Ann Holohan describes her reaction to the threat of a possible malignant breast tumor and the doctor's announcement of the need for a biopsy:

I got up, struggled to preserve normality (this seemed enormously important) and was astonished to hear myself asking mundane questions about admission procedures for tomorrow. He opened the door and still in a state of utter turmoil, I walked into the street. It seemed incredible that nothing had changed—the sun was still shining, the road sweeper gathering the leaves. I sat in my car, and with the conventional constraints removed, immense waves of panic engulfed me. I drove blindly home and recall very little of the actual journey. I felt this alien, pathological change was inexorable, gone was the reassuring external cause of my symptoms. Yet clearly I was no "sicker" than before my consultation. All that had changed was the possibility of a medical label for my symptom.

(1977, 87–88)

As it turned out, Holohan did not have cancer; the tumor was benign. But the possibility and the meaning of that possibility for her elicited psychological and physical reactions far beyond the lesion, which was not producing any noticeable symptoms at the time.

Innumerable cancer patients have shared Holohan's experience. Many cultural influences contribute to patient reactions, including perceptions of vulnerability, what people know and do not know about cancer, others' attitudes toward the disease, degree of trust in the doctor's diagnostic and treatment abilities, and perception of the disruption of one's life, including the threat to end it. In addition, the patient would have to consider the cost of unguaranteed survival—in financial terms, personal time lost, pain and suffering, and the effects on family. He or she would have to deal with deciding, with doctors and others, on whether and how to treat the cancer, as well.

In terms of meaning, then, we are dealing with two typologies, both of which may be socially and culturally constructed: the patient's expectations and experience of personal and social effects on her life (**illness**), and the physician's experience of treating a concrete biological entity (**disease**). To say that a disease is "socially constructed" does not necessarily deny the biological reality of the disease (Lock 1988). It does, however, recognize that the meaning of the illness for both healer and patient derives from its historical, cultural, and individual, as well as biological context (Brandt 1991, 204).

It has generally been assumed that diagnoses and decision making on the part of physicians takes place in a clinically autonomous environment, is objectively based on signs and symptoms, and is isolated from the social milieu. In an extensive literature review of the role of social structure in clinical decision making, however, Clark, Potter, and McKinlay (1991) noted the influence of preconceived ideas of providers that, for example, result in the underdetection of coronary heart disease in women. This situation may be changing, as more research shows that estrogen is not as protective as previously thought. The Framingham study, one of the most extensive studies ever to be undertaken in relation to heart disease, using age-adjusted data, showed that women have nearly 50 percent more silent heart attacks, have higher case fatality rates, and present with more advanced or severe heart disease than men (Clark, Potter, and McKinlay 1991, 862). Thus, the researchers concluded that "research designs should now go further in specifying the linkages between physicians' thinking, their interaction with patients, and the wider social structure" (862).

Brown provides one way of doing so in his "sociology of diagnosis" (1995), a typology of conditions and definitions. "Routine conditions," covering the vast majority, are easiest to diagnose, least conflictual, and involve primarily an adjustment and adaptation on the part of the patient, who may reject the diagnosis due to its disruptive potential. "Medicalized definitions" involve conditions that are generally nonmedical where biomedical definitions are applied. Medical labeling here may be a form of social control or professional expansion or may be a source of legitimation for many vague conditions such as chronic fatigue or pain syndromes. "Contested definitions" are those that may be widely accepted, but with no accompanying applied clinical medical definition, such as in the case of chemical contamination of military personnel during the Persian Gulf War. This hesitancy for medical confirmation may arise out of rigid diagnostic criteria, opposition to lay involvement in diagnoses, and fear of political and economic consequences. Finally, "potentially medicalized definitions" are those conditions not currently medicalized, but that may be so in the future, such as genetic predispositions, identified through screening. These conditions are not in themselves medical conditions, and they may never become such (40–42). Nevertheless, "these screening approaches wind up defining as pathology the genetic makeup, rather than the disease that may arise" (42). Possible consequences are workplace exclusion policies, where the victim is blamed for a predisposition, and exclusion from insurance coverage.

BIOMEDICINE AND THE DOMINANT CAPITALIST CULTURE

One of biomedicine's early roots was the tradition of service to suffering humanity, an ideal value strongly supported in the United States. The developing structure of the American biomedical system, however, supported and was more consistent with the values of capitalist enterprise, as we have seen in the struggle for status and control, competition for markets, and political maneuvering of vested capitalist interests. The basic environment was one of marketplace medicine, where clinical services were sold to the patient for a fee by a practitioner in private practice.

The capitalist connection was even more apparent when biomedicine, in the 1960s, responded with fierce resistance to the implementation of the government-sponsored programs of Medicare and Medicaid, which provide funds for care for the aged and the poor, respectively. As Milford O. Rouse, a former president of the AMA, stated at the time: "We are faced with the concept of health care as a right rather than a privilege. . . . What is our philosophy? It is the faith in private enterprise. We can, therefore, concentrate our attention on the single obligation to protect the American way of life. That way can be described in one word: Capitalism" (quoted in Montagu 1969, E-13).

The seeming contradiction of service versus profit underwrites one of the perennial questions facing the medical profession: If the free-enterprise system is incapable of providing care for all those who require it and care is to be conceived of as a right rather than a privilege, then how, and by whom, is it to be delivered and financed? The 1960s introduction of the Medicare and Medicaid programs was a recognition that rising costs and restricted access required government intervention.

Although the AMA denounced both Medicare and Medicaid as threats to private enterprise and "the American way," Medicare was ultimately rationalized as acceptable through the input of Social Security payments and inclusion of payment of physicians' fees. Medicaid, however, because it was directed to the poor and devolved to the states for budgeting and administration, was underfunded—and therefore much less lucrative. It was also seen as a less legitimate form of public assistance in a capitalist society, and physician participation was far more limited (Starr 1982).

In the 1960s, the growing emphasis on health care as a right, as well as the perspective that illness could be and was socially engendered, involved conceptual shifts, and motivated some government intervention—but it did not demand structural changes. Renee Fox wrote that discussions regarding the destratification of the physician's role and the concept of national health insurance in the 1970s actually reaffirmed the traditional American values of equality, independence, self-reliance, universalism, distributive justice, solidarity, reciprocity, and individual and community responsibility (1977, 21).

Still, Fox predicted little change in the overall structure of health care, noting that in spite of trends toward increased appreciation of the influences on health of personal behavior, greater use of nonphysician professionals, and greater emphasis on prevention, "none of these trends implies that what we have called cultural demedicalization will take place." By this, Fox meant that health, illness, and medicine would, in future, remain central preoccupations of the society, and that they would maintain the "social, ethical, and existential significance they have acquired" (1977, 21). Thus far, this seems to be the case. Biomedicine as a part of culture essentially incorporates, supports, and reflects both the ideals and realities of society in its philosophies and functions.

Even science itself, the foundation on which biomedicine rests, reflects social realities and is open to cultural analysis.

HOW "SCIENTIFIC" IS SCIENCE?

As Dossey (1982) observes, "Although science demands proof that observations made by one observer be observable by other observers using the same methods, it is by no means clear that, even when confronted with identical phenomena, different observers will report identical observations" (9). If the content of medical science was unaffected by culture, this would not be the case.

When Payer (1996) investigated biomedical practice in Great Britain, Germany, France, and the United States, she found many differences. The British prescribed fewer drugs in general than the French or Germans. The patient in Great Britain was about one-half as likely as an American to have surgery of any kind. Daily vitamin requirements were smaller. British doctors were more reluctant than American ones to diagnose someone as "sick" based upon similar signs and symptoms.

In Germany, low blood pressure was a condition requiring treatment to raise it, unlike the United States where it was and is treated as a "nondisease" indicative of long life. Germans prescribed far fewer antibiotics and far more heart drugs than the other nationalities; they consider the heart to be greatly affected by emotions, rather than a pump that can be replaced.

French biomedicine concentrated on building up the physical and mental constitution (termed "terrain") with vitamins, tonics, diet, and exercise, rather than aggressively attacking the disease with drugs and medications. The French performed very few hysterectomies compared to the United States. Treatment for psychiatric problems was likely to be a visit to a government-approved spa, a long sick leave, or a "sleep cure."

Finally, the practice of scientific medicine in the United States was—and generally is—highly aggressive, and directed toward attacking the lesion, or disease; the body is considered a machine to be "fixed." Even psychoanalysis in the United States was not concerned with emotions, but "rearranges things inside the mind the way surgery rearranges things inside the body" (Janet Malcomb, quoted in Payer 1996, 150). Payer added that "anything that cannot fit into the machine model of the body, or be quantified, is often denied not only quantification, but even existence" (151).

These major differences in perception and use of medical knowledge and content may be waning as medicine becomes globalized (often Americanized; e.g., Watters 2010). Nonetheless, differences that do persist reflect, among other things, basic cultural values. The French highly value having children and the aesthetics of appearance. The Germans, although characterized as authoritarian, are influenced by nineteenth-century Romanticism and see themselves as emotional, accommodating the various facets of efficiency, spirituality, and nature—hence the focus on the heart. The English practice an "economy" in their medicine, partly due to the payment incentives for doctors, but also because, it is suggested, the British are taught to deny the body. They are expected to exhibit stoicism and maintain a "stiff upper lip" (Payer 1996).

In the United States, the practice of an aggressive, heroic style of medicine, where doing something is always better than doing nothing, fits well into the national psyche (mind-set or direction of thinking). The compatibility of heroic medicine with American values was noted long ago by Oliver Wendell Holmes, who wrote:

> How could a people. . . . which insists in sending out yachts and horses and boys to out-sail, out-run, out-fight, and checkmate all the rest of creation; how could such a people be content with any but "heroic" practice? What wonder that the Stars and Stripes wave over doses of ninety grains of sulphate of quinine, or that the American eagle screams with delight to see three drachms of calomel given at a single mouthful?
>
> (Holmes 1888, 193)

These early values and approaches are still dominant. Some treatment decisions have become even more "heroic" with the growth of technological possibilities, such as keeping comatose people alive on respirators; when there is no hope of recovery or even improvement, such treatment may be interpreted as totally inappropriate (Johnson 1996, 20).

The meanings of scientific findings are hotly debated by physicians and scientists alike as they attempt to understand and interpret medical information, using their educational and experiential resources, including cultural factors of which they may be totally unaware. Some recent cases in point involve how to treat breast cancer and whether the removal of the entire breast with underlying muscle is the best approach; whether more expensive and dangerous bypass surgery is better in heart disease than less invasive angioplasty, which widens arteries, or even just diet and exercise; whether to circumcise male infants; and whether to treat depression with strong and some-times dangerous medications with unknown side effects.

Both doctor and patient are dealing with odds and a cost-benefit problem, making absolute decisions based on relative perspectives (Lock 1993, 337–40; Mack and Ross 1989). To the physician, the risk may be worth the benefit, but to the patient, it may not—or vice versa. There-fore, these decisions must be based upon personal and cultural meanings and implications as well as on whatever scientific information is available, as interpreted by the physician and considered by the patient.

The problem is compounded, because scientific results may also be confusing and subject to different interpretations. For example, Mack and Ross (1989), after performing an extensive risk-benefit analy-sis of estrogen use (discussed by Lock 1993), recommended "prudent" use of estrogen without other hormones. Most physicians, however, at the time recommended that combined therapy should always be used (reported in Coney 1994). Similar discrepancies still abound, such as in contrary recommendations regarding mammograms, pediatric male circumcision, and various types of medical testing, such as for prostate disease. In each case, differing subcultures of the profession are at odds.

BIOMEDICINE AS CULTURE

Rather than being a culture-free system, biomedicine, as we have seen, may be viewed as one element or approach within a larger cultural system. It may also be examined as a cultural system itself (Hahn 1995), however unsystematic it may in some ways be. One way of characteriz-ing a medical system would be to include the elements of illness, people, environment, resources, and beliefs (Gesler 1991, 21). A medical system would include types of illness present; socially sanctioned healers and the means, method, and content of their training; a structured means of delivery of care; designated locations for care delivery; a means of financing or paying for care; philosophies and ideas about health and illness; and all the links, interactions, inputs, and outputs between and among elements (Robertson and Heagarty 1975). These elements can also be broken down according to their characteristics and vary from medical system to medical system, time to time, and place to place. The interrelationships of elements, however, are directed to the purpose of prevention, cure, and control of illness.

The system of biologically based medical care involves a technical language, a central belief and value system, rituals, and symbols different from those of the general society. Johnson refers to this as a "medical paradigm" (model), which can be compared to other medical paradigms such as that of Hippocrates (1996, 18). There can be many variations within the paradigmatic structure. The doctor-patient relationship, for example, may vary according to patient population, setting of care, medical diagnosis, and so forth; and some physicians may be more oriented within the biological, psychological, or social perspectives.

The special language of biomedicine gives clinical meaning to disease through labeling. A diagnosis of infection with *Clostridium tetani*, or tetanus, for example, indicates to the physician that a deep puncture wound allowed anaerobic bacteria to enter the bloodstream of the patient; the tetanospasmin in the toxin binds to the ganglioside membranes of nerve synapses, blocking the release of the inhibitory transmitter from the nerve terminals, thereby causing a generalized tonic spasticity upon which intermittent tonic convulsions are usually superimposed (*The Merck Manual* 1982, 113–14). This, of course, means little or nothing to the patient who suffers and whose ideas of cause and effect may be quite different and include anything from punishment for past sins to plain bad luck.

In many instances, the language of biomedicine is inadequate for discussing what ails us. Suffering comes in many forms and varies across cultures and historical epochs; it may be caused by loss, defeat, and social injustice, in contrast to causes located within the body. The discourse of our biomedical culture (for example, the disease concept) is thus ill suited for representing and comprehending some major forms of human suffering (Shweder 1991, with reference to Kleinman 1986b).

THE EXTENSION OF MEDICAL CULTURE AND SOCIAL CONTROL

The label of "disease," which implies submission to the official medical system designed to address it (Parsons 1951), may not be adequate in addressing suffering. But it has been increasingly applied to a number of human conditions and behaviors defined as **deviant** (i.e., different or apart from the norm).

Since deviance may generally be seen as willful or unwillful, crime and illness may be viewed as alternate designations for deviance (Conrad and Schneider 1992, 36). Deviance not viewed as willful is seen as amenable to help and treatment, rather than as criminal behavior to be punished. Through the process of **medicalization**, physicians define in medical terms what may have been considered a personal or social problem and propose medical treatment as an appropriate solution. When illness is the designation, medicine becomes the agent of social control. In the case of chemical dependency, for example, "medicine replaces or collaborates with the criminal justice system" (Brown 1995, 41).

Alcoholism provides a good example. As a medical problem, alcoholism is labeled a disease over which the sufferer has little or no control and is treated with medications and even personal psychiatric counseling, often at inpatient alcohol treatment facilities. Demedicalization would occur when the problem is once again viewed as personal deviance or human weakness to be addressed by education or strong social sanctions and possibly incarceration as punishment.

Other medicalized areas include childbirth (discussed in Chapter 3), behavioral manifestations such as hyperactivity and aggressiveness, sleep disorders, "low" sex drive, and even male baldness. One example of a historical medicalized condition would be women's enjoyment of sexuality. In some places during the nineteenth century, such enjoyment was labeled a disease and was treated, sometimes by even removing the clitoris. Today in some cultures, due to the changing view of women as full participants in society, with a right to recognize the sexual side of their nature, it is considered unhealthy if a woman fails to enjoy her sexuality (A. Johnson 1996). She may now be treated with hormones or counseling for "frigidity" in order to regain her "sexual potential."

Even the elderly are subject to medicalization. For instance, McLean's work with nursing home staff and residents shows how resident elders' refusal to tolerate demeaning or dehumanizing treatment, often demonstrated by withdrawal or noncooperative and sometimes disruptive behavior, is cast by providers as medically rooted rather than socioculturally generated and therefore treated with pharmaceutical means (2007).

Current U.S. culture is quite receptive to the process of medicalization. Capitalism allows for the creation of new and highly profitable markets, and medicalization has the potential for creating new markets through expanded definitions of social and personal problems. Thus, the medical conceptions of deviance in American society have "a cultural resonance both with dominant values and the organizational apparatus to promote and sustain them, creating a fertile environment for medicalization" (Conrad and Schneider 1992, 265).

It is doubtful that the process of medicalization could occur to the extent identified if the appeal were not related to cultural values and norms. For example, drinking has generally been tacitly accepted in our society, particularly among males. It has also been viewed as a norm, a symbol of sociability, recreation, and escape from the stresses of life. "Holding" one's liquor has also been a mark of masculinity. Once a drinker has progressed to the point of becoming an alcoholic, medicalization relieves the drinker of personal responsibility and provides a socially acceptable therapy for recovery. The label makes the problem less devastating for both the drinker and her or his family.

The appeal of medically preventing, halting, or reversing hair loss in males, which is not a medical problem in itself, can be seen as relating to high social values placed on youth. Loss of hair signifies the process of aging and loss of currently defined physical attractiveness. Hair loss as a medical problem can be addressed by medical treatment. Recall the advertisements to "see your doctor" because "there *is* hope," sponsored by a pharmaceutical producer of a drug to stimulate new hair growth. The tenor of the appeal is that of curing a disease condition rather than as a cosmetic appeal to vanity, which in American culture is as unmanly as a receding hairline.

The social sciences have produced numerous attacks on this extension of medical labeling. The medicalization of American society is interpreted as a type of "medical imperialism" that extends medical authority and power over wider aspects of American life (cf. Conrad and Schneider 1992). However, in some cases such as alcoholism, the medical profession may be only marginally involved. Treatment is not required for designation as a medical condition. In addition, some conditions that were once considered as medical problems have actually been "demedicalized," including masturbation and homosexuality. Further, although public tolerance for discomfort has decreased, there is less access to care. The lack of trust in the medical profession and reduction of utilization may act to limit medicalization (Conrad 2000, 322–23). As Armstrong points out, "The future of medicine in its various forms can only be analyzed in the context of a society of which it is part, and with which it has reciprocal relations" (1989, 130).

Indeed, a new paradigm for medicalization—"geneticization"—has recently emerged in response to advances in our knowledge of the mapping of the human genome, termed "geneticization" of human problems (Lippman 1991). As Conrad suggests, "How much genetics will influence the direction and degree of medicalization is not yet known. To the extent that scientific research and new paradigms influence the definition and treatment of human problems, genetics, along with neuroscience and psychopharmacology, will be a significant factor (331).

DOCTOR-PATIENT, PROVIDER-CONSUMER

The physician-patient relationship is generally taken as the central element in health care (Glass 1996; Hahn 1995). This relationship has long been a topic of study for both medical sociology and anthropology, and includes factors of trust, communication, decision making, and power.

According to the cultural ideals of biomedicine, the physician possesses the technical abilities, within limits, of alleviating the patient's suffering, treating illness, and preserving life. The patient, on the other hand, is threatened with pain, disability, and the possible end of existence and must rely on the doctor's knowledge, skill, and moral and ethical behavior. This requires a great deal of trust on the part of the patient. That trust is not always easily established.

There are numerous historical examples of physicians withholding diagnostic information from patients and divulging as little information on patients' conditions as considered possible or prudent. Even Hippocrates advised concealing information from patients. The rationale included patient inability to understand or interpret medical information. This rationale has not entirely disappeared today, but numerous social forces have altered attitudes and approaches. Better-educated patients, the wealth of medical and health care information available to the public, increasing interest in and practice of self-care in terms of diet and exercise, the growing problems of chronic illness, increased reliance on technological means of diagnosis and treatment—all have created pressures for change and a more "patient-centered" medicine.

The shift to **patient-centered care**, described by Laine and Davidoff (1996), deemphasizes the idea of compliance and stresses information sharing, shared decision making, and other forms of patient participation and patient-provider partnership; it does, however, allow for some diversity and selectivity in assessing what patients really prefer or want to know. Patients coming from other cultural backgrounds (or with particular kinds of previous experience) may not expect or even want detailed medical information about their conditions. For example, in Japan that information is commonly withheld.

A series of letters in the *Journal of the American Medical Association* (1996, 107–10) focused on the Navajo concept of *hozho*, which prohibits speaking directly of negative issues such as possible complications of surgery, adverse effects of medication, or even death, since to do so makes them more likely to happen. Responses to the difficulty included comments that "refusing to give them the facts about their condition and possible treatment because they belong to a particular ethnic group is not only unethical but absurd" (108). But they also included suggestions from practitioners who treat Navajo patients and find that use of third-person plural in discussions works very well and that "in general, Navajo patients quickly identify this good faith effort made by the practitioner and seem to be more willing and able to understand the 'negatives' in medicine." This view also recognizes that "such culturally sensitive communication can lead to more informed decisions and better outcomes" (108). Thus a more patient-centered approach would seem, by definition, to consider the issues of cultural sensitivity and patient expectations and preferences, as part of patients' rights.

The battle for patient-centered care is not easily won. In the past, before the increase in focus on scientific therapeutics, doctors were encouraged to let the patient talk as a means of therapeutic intervention and included the doctor's respectful and undivided attention, rather than "interrogation" (Shorter 1985, 157–64). But in the 1990s, citing the growing tensions between the medical science and medical art (care), including strains due to rapid changes in practice economics such as specialization and technological advance, and the way that the biomedical model ignores psychosocial factors and isolates physicians from their patients as persons, the patient-physician relationship seemed to some to be "under siege" (Glass 1996, 147).

In discussing this "siege," Glass (1996) cited a "new paradigm": **evidence-based medicine**, also known as evidence-based practice, which initially emerged as an alternative to the rise of organizationally imposed restrictions on what doctors could do, and as a way to manage the proliferation of clinical literature (Sobo 2009a, 153–55). Evidence-based medicine emphasizes the *critical* assessment of clinical science in diagnosis and points out that if the "critical" is emphasized, then science need not separate doctor and patient. Starting from the patient, the provider formulates a structured, answerable question and goes to the evidence base to answer that question (Lipman 2000, 561; Sackett et al. 1996). Physicians thus use the best that science has to offer in formulating care plan options, but not at the expense of an acknowledgment of psychosocial issues or the uniqueness of each patient as a person. A later outgrowth of this focus has been the use of evidence-based clinical practice guidelines for diagnosis and care plan design.

While there is some fear today that this approach might mean denying care to people who, from a statistical perspective, may not benefit, evidence-based medicine ideally stresses consideration, empathy, and compassion, and entails patient involvement. It rejects the idea of organizationally mandated one-size-fits-all clinical algorithm or guideline application. Nonetheless, it still is located well within the biomedical paradigm; it does not broaden the "evidence" to include the sociocultural issues outside the biomedical culture that are so vital to communication and understanding. Nor does it reduce the need for developing intuition and clinical judgment.

The strain of health care economics also threatens to intervene in the doctor-patient relationship because of intensifying patient needs, and costs inherent in exchange of fee for service. With the direct entry of corporate entities into the health care field and the rise of managed care in the 1980s, the discourse of medicine began to take on the language of the marketplace. Managed care, and the clinical audit systems whose emergence underwrote it, assumed that factory management strategies that focused on reducing overlap, unnecessary variation, and overuse, as well as business valuation measures, could be applied to health care (see Sobo 2009a, Chapter 8). Patients became "clients" or "consumers"; physicians, nurses, and so on became "providers." Incentives changed, as medical care became a "product" to be purchased. Major and persisting concerns fostered by this shift include less time spent with each patient, loss of physician autonomy in clinical decision making, loss of continuity in patient care, loss of patient trust, and the adversarial and ethical problems that arise when decisions are driven by financial concerns rather than by the best interests of the patient (Glass 1996, 1296).

The trend toward patient-centered care and evidence-based practice may prove to offset some of the negative influences of marketplace medicine, provided that evidentiary standards be broadened beyond the typical clinical trials type of data, which illuminates a treatment's efficacy under experimental conditions but does little to enrich our understanding about effectiveness in real-life settings (Sobo 2009a, Chapter 8). Another issue to be resolved relates to the previously discussed need to consider patients as part of a family or household unit (see Chapter 2) rather than treating each as an isolated individual. Patient-centered care is in reality "family-centered care" and that the doctor-patient dyad must be expanded to include family and household members.

Paradoxically, these trends may actually be supported by consumerism, since new consumers of health care are more informed, wish to have their own preferences considered, and have become more accustomed to questioning physician authority. Patient-centered care may also help address the problem of malpractice suits against physicians since it has been shown that various physician behavior such as disrespect and devaluing or ignoring patients' questions and perspectives are positively associated with malpractice claims (Laine and Davidoff 1996; also see Beckman et al. 1994; Forster, Wchwartz, and DeRenzo 2002).

WHERE TO NOW?

Managed care and corporate involvement in medicine mean that providers are subject to policy and managerial constraints that entail conflicts of interest, divided loyalties, and ethical dilemmas. Providers are expected to conform to the rules and policies of the managed care organization, which may be in conflict with the patient's welfare and the clinician's role as patient advocate (Waitzkin 2000).

Paradoxically, corporate focus on the bottom line could also ultimately serve to bring doctors and patients back together. Some in the 1990s predicted that, in the role of patient advocate, physicians may join with patients to "hold third parties accountable to their claims that high quality of care, rather than purely low cost, is their mission" (Laine and Davidoff 1996, 155). Further, the base of biomedical knowledge has expanded to include more research on social issues as well as the perspectives and concerns of patients. There still is a long way to go, but inroads have definitely been made.

In the next chapter, we discuss the changing face of health care today. These include ethical dilemmas, the growing pressures and need for system reform, and culturally based resistance to that reform.

FOR DISCUSSION

1. Discuss early medical care in the United States. How did it reflect medical pluralism and a multicultural population?

2. What factors, other than scientific advances, have contributed to the development of the American biomedical system? Characterize the American biomedical system in terms of its consistency with the dominant culture.

3. Considering the influences of technology, managed care, and the changing doctor-patient relationship, what predictions might we make regarding biomedicine's future evolution and development?

CHAPTER 6

Reforming Medicine

GOAL: Explore the impact of science and technology as agents of change in the health care system; become familiar with related arguments, issues, models, and systems.

GOAL: Understand the relationships of change in technologies, medical progress, patient needs, and provider dilemmas to the social structure and reform of the health care system.

GOAL: Examine the nature of culturally based social, economic, and political resistance to health care reform.

GOAL: Acknowledge globalization's impact on health care concerns and delivery.

A society's commitment to health care reflects some of its most basic values about what it is to be a member of the human community. Therefore, it can be argued that society has an ethical obligation to ensure equitable access to health services by making that care a basic social right. This is because of health care's special importance to society in relieving suffering, preventing premature death, and restoring the ability to function to the people who live in it.

(Cockerham 2010, 329)

Although change often produces anxiety and even fear, particularly in those who have a vested interest in the status quo, change is inevitable. The agents of that change include technological and scientific advancement, economic conditions, availability and scarcity of resources, cultural mix and diversity, population increase or decline, social structure, environmental change, and political leadership.

As the dominant medical system, biomedicine has often been highly resistant to change, partly because of its fragmented nature, but also because of more complex issues of power, control, and the economic structure (see Imershein 1981). Changes have generally occurred only when seen as necessary "fixes." Large-scale programs such as Medicare and Medicaid introduced by the government as a response to critical needs were at first strongly opposed by various groups, including physicians, but were ultimately absorbed into the system. Indeed, to some, the interventional origin of these programs is not even a dim memory: In a recent reform-related town hall meeting covered by the *New York Times*, "a man stood up and told Representative Bob Inglis to 'keep your government hands off my Medicare'" (Krugman 2009).

Other changes introduced by the government and others have included the development of health maintenance organizations, the emergence of new allied and adjunct paraprofessionals as well as new medical specialties (including family practice), and development of programs of health education and promotion along with new specialties such as health educators. These changes mostly affected the way health care was delivered, but failed to address rising costs, growing demand and limited supply, the growing numbers of citizens without health insurance, and their inability to afford and have access to pharmaceuticals and other expensive treatments. The system itself remained fairly intact.

Changes also did little to address cultural issues. Things are changing, but still, questions regarding quality of care and disparities within the population, cultural sensitivity of providers and educators, cost-effective care and care delivery across disparate groups, coordinated care, and a continuum of care for individual patients over the life cycle are only a few culturally related areas yet to be effectively addressed in a rapidly changing society.

One very important area that has become particularly notable because of technological advances and growing treatment options for some but not all populations, is bioethics. Bioethics also has yet to successfully address cultural diversity and the difficulties this poses for developing treatment standards, for decision making, and for reducing the serious disparities that still exist in health status and health care delivery (Pamies and Nsiah-Kumi 2009).

BIOETHICS IN CULTURAL CONTEXT

Having a code of ethics is one criterion for professional status. Ethical decision making, however, has always been a part of the profession of biomedicine, whether those decisions were made jointly by patients and doctors, doctors alone, or as accepted policies in health care institutions.

Early Western biomedical ethics reflected, among other things, the Hippocratic Oath, which exhorts physicians, if they cannot help, to at least "do no harm." Ethics were located within the context of possibilities (i.e., existing knowledge and the boundaries of the physician's role). The moral imperative to "do no harm" recognizes that harm is possible. As previously noted, the profit (versus service) orientation was also recognized early on, along with its temptations and possibilities. Ethical codes, then, not only can be a measure of professionalism, but can serve as a means of social control over "unethical" behavior, using the threat of loss of professional identity and status.

With the greater capacities of modern medicine to do good, the potential to do harm is also increased, even when unintentional. "Harm" is not an easy concept to define, in view of the fact that medicine must often harm in order to heal, as in chemotherapy for cancer. Also, what is harm to one may not be harm to another, as in invasive or painful treatment to maintain life when no other benefit or improvement can be derived.

Bioethics (ethics applied to biomedicine) also cannot be viewed as acultural, or outside of the influences of culture. The main stuff of bioethics concerns human values and beliefs that reflect or are translated into social structure and activity. Because Western bioethics is oriented within the Western value system and has been basically guided by principles of beneficence, justice, nonmalfeasance (doing no harm), and individual autonomy (Kissell 2009, 60–61), the biomedical health care system has been guided by those same values. This leaves no recognition of ethical systems that reflect other worldviews and other cultural orientations. In addition, the Western value system contains its own contradictions (Ratliff 1996).

The wide disparities apparent in access to health care in the United States, for example, reflect the paradox in our values and beliefs as a society. As Williams noted early on (1970, Chapter 1), our dominant values include humanitarianism and support of the "underdog" and equality for all. If health care is defined as a right, then we have a duty to provide health care to all members of the society. However, it is often argued that there is no intrinsic right to health care. Thus there is no social obligation or duty to provide health care to those who cannot purchase it. By the same token, it could be argued that no one would then have an intrinsic right to use the freeway systems, to police and fire protection, to safe food and drinking water, to education, or to any other public services now available to all.

Western bioethics also has been criticized as too focused on the individual and his or her autonomy. In some cultures, such as among some Asian or Hispanic groups, family, community, and interdependence are much more important: Individuals may not make decisions for or about themselves without consulting family or group members. Also, as Ratliff (1996) points out, because we are interconnected, whatever affects some affects all; and therefore there is a social responsibility incumbent on all of us. Health care not made available to people who cannot pay, for example, may result in spread of illness and disease, or of reducing the workforce and reducing production when workers are ill and unable to work. Yet many people still remain outside the system, with little or no access to health care.

To address the ethical issue of disparities in health care, Ratliff proposes a social nexus model based on the idea of a society as a ship whose members are involved in networks of interdependent relationships (nexuses). "Anything that impacts one nexus ultimately impacts all of them; that is, if one end of the social ship has sustained damage, passengers at the other end are unwise to dismiss it as not their problem (Ratliff 1996, 175). However, unless and until this sense of social responsibility becomes an integral part of the American value system, this solution remains highly unlikely. Solutions, in fact, are anything but easily agreed upon.

Bioethical debates on a myriad of ethical issues have been and are being conducted in an increasingly pluralistic, culturally fragmented, and "religiously resonant but secularized society" (Fox 1994, 49). In this atmosphere, many have felt the need for and therefore support a simplified, common, and broadly applicable way of addressing moral and ethical problems; thus, ethical issues are generally located (and generated) within the framework of the dominant culture. The ethical principles to be applied are also located within that framework. The bioethical agenda, in other words, "responds to the predominating political, economic, and value orientation of the society, which tends to reflect rather than criticize or challenge" and is more "reactive than initiatory" (Fox 1994, 49).

Some ethicists and social scientists feel that ethics discussed or considered within this "formulaic" framework have become flat, mechanical, unemotional, and formal (Fox 1994; Gustafson 1990). While there are exceptions, such discussions are often devoid of any recognition of cultural needs and diversity.

Multiculturalism presents a substantial challenge to bioethics, because cultural values of one group and ethical frameworks of another can be in conflict. Take, for instance, the question of abortion. The concepts of "human" and "person" are quite distinct in many non-Western societies. The rights accorded to persons may be quite different from those accorded to humans. In some societies, after biological birth a fetus (still so regarded by the community) must earn the status and rights of "person" by managing to survive, and gaining the vigor and health necessary for becoming a contributing member of the community; it then experiences a "social birth," which confers the rights of personhood (Morgan 1989). Most societies condemn infanticide, but only after the neonate has been recognized as a person. And as Morgan explains, "The social construction of personhood differs according to the environmental, cosmological, and historical circumstances of different societies. There can be no absolute definition of personhood isolated from a sociocultural context" (101).

Further difficulty in developing multicultural bioethics is created by the capitalist context: Bioethics, like other elements of the dominant medical system, have been subject to marketplace discourse. There is discussion of cost containment, competition, health care as a commodity subject to supply and demand, allocation of resources, economic returns from research investments, the body as private property, and questions of supply and demand for organ transplantation.

Framing ethical issues in terms of profit and loss leads away from a service orientation or one that considers health care as a social good; "furthermore, it removes the field from a conception of social justice that pays special attention to the plight of the poor, the disadvantaged, the victims of social prejudice and discrimination" (Fox 1994, 50). The service orientation, on the other hand, establishes the relevance and connection of medical ethical issues with socio-structural causes of illness and with social injustice, which includes unequal access to health care for many groups.

A panel of prominent experts sponsored by the Massachusetts Medical Society discussed U.S. health policy and health coverage in May 2008 (Morrissey 2008). Access to health care was mentioned as the most basic ethical issue of all; the panel noted that the fact that a huge number of people are not insured or are underinsured was a national shame. However, they felt that fighting the battle for health care reform on a moral-grounds argument alone (everyone deserves health care) would not work. Change, and the argument, they determined, must focus on benefits to the whole population—but the population must participate in the process.

Although consideration of costs and benefits seems to conflict with ethical considerations when many people are left out of the system due to high costs and the inability to pay, economic problems must be addressed as a subject of ethical concern. In addition, in an age of legal tangles and multiple interpretations, Supreme Court decisions, uncertainty, and fear of lawsuits—as well as confusion, human anguish, and unwillingness and inability to confront hard choices—there is a need for guidelines and the creation of some precedents, as well as recognition that resources and capabilities are finite.

Medical ethics (or bioethics) has become a respected area of expertise, with a number of established centers throughout the United States. Bioethics is a uniquely human endeavor—and as such, must reflect the diversity of human needs and perceptions. While experts can study the problems and issues and give advice and consultation, they, too, may have vested interests and agendas; they may "know," but not "see" (Lieberman 1970). Experts may determine policies and options for decision making and recommend courses of action, but the possible risks and benefits must also be assessed by those most affected—patients and their families or representatives. To this end, bioethics committees are seen as a most desirable option for consultation, reviewing cases, and offering advice to be taken or rejected by the patient or parties involved (Munson 2000). To reflect a truly multicultural input, these committees, as much as is possible, should therefore include members of varying age, gender, class, and race/ethnic groups (Lakhan et al. 2009).

The field of bioethics faces the same problems of the need for respect for diversity as those faced in biomedicine and general society. It must allow for a broader, more inclusive view of human needs and emotions while maintaining a sense of unity in ethical guidelines and flexibility in recognition of the human condition. The same applies to the biomedical model, with consideration of how to create and incorporate a more inclusive and relevant framework.

EXPANDING THE BIOMEDICAL MODEL

HOLISTIC HEALTH

The holistic health movement emerged in the early 1970s, growing out of the natural health movement of the early1900s. Holistic health incorporated a wide variety of therapeutic and alternative approaches, including humanistic and psychosomatic medicine, parapsychology, folk medicine, as well as formerly designated sectarian therapies and philosophies. However, holistic health presents an alternative medical paradigm with a different arrangement of medical practice and patient-practitioner relationships and offers some possibilities that biomedicine should consider.

Holistic practitioners constitute a highly varied group ranging from faith healers, chiropractors, and herbalists, to mainstream physicians who may use some holistic techniques. Discussing holistic health care in general is difficult at best, because practitioners and methods are so diverse. Lowenberg (1989), however, derived seven core beliefs that holistic practitioners hold in common. Generally, they view the person as a whole being situated within a total environment and see health promotion and education as vital to the healing process. The meaning of illness to holistic adherents involves all aspects of the individual—including the mental, emotional, social, spiritual, and physical.

The individual, if able, takes much responsibility for understanding his or her own illness, initiating steps to prevent illness and promote health, and actively participates in treatment. Practitioners, rather than taking the role of expert as biomedical practitioners do, become facilitators, educators, and consultants, sharing expertise with more self-directed patients. There is ideally a warm, caring setting for care delivery and more physical contact between patient and practitioner, which is seen as an important component in healing (Krieger 1984).

The last characteristic concerns an alternative worldview, or view of "consciousness." The focus on consciousness might be considered a shift of paradigms—from a reductionist, objectivist model to a more all-inclusive, holistic one (Dossey 1982).

The holistic health model fills gaps and provides alternative explanations for problems not addressed by the biomedical model. Nevertheless, the holistic model itself also contains a number of problems and limitations that must be recognized—particularly in the area of self-responsibility and doctor-patient relationships.

Making the individual primarily responsible for his or her own health and illness puts the patient in charge, but can lead to "blaming the victim" when an individual remains or becomes ill. It can also be lethal. One 44-year-old with malignant melanoma, a deadly skin cancer, tried mental imagery to effect a cure, but "when it failed to arrest the disease, she began to blame herself. She was pained by the possibility that her own psychological defects brought on the disease and precluded her ability to cure herself" (Cassileth, cited in Williams 1993, 78).

Dossey cautions that the holistic insistence on the concept of individual self is inconsistent with the true meaning of "holism," which involves interconnections with all other individuals and environments. "The holistic movement," notes Dossey, "commits the same failure as the traditional system of medical care by placing primacy on the *objectivity* of health care" and both paradigms are still located in a similar worldview of cause and effect (1982, 214; italics in original).

Similarities between the holistic and the biomedical model also are suggested by Berliner and Salmon (1980) in patterns of fee-for-service entrepreneurial practice, knowledge sold to consumers as a commodity, elitist and sexist behavior of practitioners, availability of services to those who can pay, clear separation between patients and practitioners, and disregard of larger societal factors as causing and contributing to disease (143). As suggested by Baer, holism as a model is limited, stressing mind-body connections but lacking connections of mind-body-society (2001, 189).

Research on outcomes of holistic treatment has often been contradictory and inconclusive. Incorporation and integration with biomedical treatments would seem to hold the most promise, but much more research on outcomes of holistic approaches alone, in contrast to and in combination with biomedical therapies is needed. If this is to take place, however, Watkins notes, "these systems either have to be proven effective by allopathic [biomedical] mechanisms, or *allopathy has to accept that they may work via mechanisms that are foreign to the present biomedical model*" (1996, 55, emphasis added).

While allopathic physicians have been slow to recognize or accept the holistic model or holistic therapies, nursing has not. This is perhaps due to the fact that, in hospitals and long-term care facilities, nurses spend more time with patients than doctors. Nursing has been at the forefront in recognition of the need for a multicultural and more holistic approach to care and caregiving.

The American Nurses Association's Code for Nurses provides the framework for culturally sensitive care in which nurses become the liaison between patient and provider. Nurses are to practice with compassion and respect for every individual without consideration of "social or economic status, personal attributes, or the nature of health problems" (Ford 2009, 91). This is especially important because research has shown that many physicians are influenced in diagnosis and treatment by their own biases regarding racial and ethnic stereotypes, as well as by shorter provider visits based on expectations of insurance companies (91).

NURSING'S CULTURE CARE THEORY

Nurses are the providers who deal most continuously with the pain and suffering of patients in their care. Thus, although trained within the scientific biomedical paradigm, they have long recognized both the needs and benefits of a dual approach; nursing has therefore been in the forefront of promoting cultural sensitivity in health care. In the 1950s, the Transcultural Nursing Society's founder Madeleine Leininger, a registered nurse who had done doctoral work in anthropology, began to develop the "culture care diversity and universality" (or "culture care") theory (Leininger 2002).

Largely due to her fieldwork in New Guinea, Leininger recognized that people culturally differ in the ways they view professional nursing and patient care needs. She was aware that cultural factors influence patient behavior, as well as well-being and outcome of care, and recognized the related need for nurses to consider both emic (local or insider) and etic (in this case, science's) views in treating and caring for their patients. She also distinguished between humanistic caring and scientific caring—relating the first to subjective feelings, experiences, and interactions, and the second to those activities and judgments that have been tested or are based on verified and quantified knowledge related to specific variables.

In 1975 Leininger developed the Sunrise Model or Sunrise Enabler— a graphic conceptualization meant to help nurses visualize ways to implement "culture care." The figure, a semicircle resting on a baseline horizon like a sun rising, depicts in its spokes or rays holistic facets and dimensions of caring for patients in a culturally sensitive way, highlighting "world view, religion, kinship, cultural values, economics, technology, language, ethnohistory, and environmental factors that are predicted to explain and influence culture care" (Leininger 1993, 26–27; 2002). Leininger has continued to develop implementation and teaching tools in her role as transcultural nursing's founder and leader.

As nursing has become more professionalized and is subjected to the same commercializing forces as those faced by physicians, the popularity of Leininger's idea of "culture care" across health care professions might be seen as a reaction to the concomitant organizational de-emphasis on and withdrawal of support for *caring*. Although certainly most applicable in nursing, due to intense patient and family contact, the lessons of culture care are relevant to the medical profession, to physicians, and to all who provide care to the ill and suffering. (In Chapter 7 we explore the evolution of the cultural emphasis through the cultural competence movement that later emerged.)

THE BIOPSYCHOSOCIAL MODEL

In response to the reductionist biomedical model, George Engel (1977) advanced another model that went beyond the strictly physical: the **biopsychosocial model**. The actual impetus for the generation of this model came from within medicine itself, and its construction reflected the recognition that in order to provide effective medical care, the psychosocial factors would have to be addressed. Engel's model appeared originally as a "psychiatric" perspective with the ultimate goal of integration into all biomedical education (Lyng 1990).

Engel recognized a tremendous advantage in the biomedical approach, but also saw the limitations that were reflected in public dissatisfaction with the growing dehumanization apparent in biomedical practice, as well as a multitude of problems such as unnecessary hospitalization, overuse of drugs, unnecessary surgery, and inappropriate diagnostic testing (1977, 134). The biopsychosocial model was also constructed on the basis of systems theory. It provided a framework, an integrated hierarchy, for the separate domains of health—the biological, psychological, and social—as a means of identifying their relationships and, thereby, the holistic nature of medicine.

Engel recognized that social factors could influence the existence and perceptions of disease; however, he still accorded biomedicine the top status in the hierarchy and advocated the inclusion of the psychosocial dimensions of illness, "soundly based on scientific principles" (1977, 135). Therefore, rather than providing an inclusive model, the biopsychosocial model essentially co-opts the psychosocial under the bio. Systems theory neutralizes the challenges of alternatives by simply presenting them as different levels of explanation of the same phenomena; thus they remain compatible with the biomedical model (Armstrong 1987, 1214). The reductionist model of biomedicine and the primacy of science is thus not only maintained, but strengthened.

The "new model," argues Armstrong, is "simply the old one with a gloss" (1987, 1217). In addition, Armstrong cites the sociological research of recent years that challenges many of the assumptions of science and the biomedical perspective: the statistical definition of "normal" and "proper functioning," the social definitions and concepts of disease, and the social, economic, and political influences that played a large part in the rise of biomedical dominance—all of which are ignored by Engel.

From Armstrong's perspective, the biopsychosocial model will neither deconstruct nor reconstruct the world of illness. On the other hand, the model might provide a means to shift the biomedical perspective. It has opened the door to consideration of psychological and social dimensions of the patient as person. If, for example, in conjunction with other growing expressions of the limitations of a purely biomedical approach, the biopsychosocial model encourages exploration of alternative structures and possibilities, it can help provide an expansion rather than a confirmation of the reductionist model through emphasis on connections of mind, body, and social milieu. In fact, it already has done so.

EMERGING INNOVATIONS AND EXPERIMENTS IN HEALTH CARE DELIVERY

The United States health care system is changing. The boom in information technology, for example, has led to emergent shifts. We have already seen this in the development of evidence-based medicine, which relies heavily on electronic publication databases (see Chapter 5). But information technology had other effects as well.

THE INTERNET

Information technology is changing health care delivery faster than many people can comprehend (see Baker et. al. 2003; Brownstein, Freifeld, and Madoff 2009; Barker, 2008). **E-health** is an umbrella term that encompasses use of the Internet, telemedicine, telehealth, and other forms of related technology. Although technology is not in itself culturally sensitive, the application of information and treatment modalities it generates can and must be culturally relevant to those it serves.

In communications, the rapidly exploding Internet now allows people to research their own and other medical problems, to chat with other people having the same problems, to learn of new discoveries and treatments, and to communicate with their physicians or caregivers—who, of course, are challenged by the increased workload and compensation problems this can entail. In any case, it is estimated that between 37 and 52 percent of Americans use the Internet each year for health-related information (Brownstein, Freifeld, and Madoff 2009). The Internet may in some ways serve as a cultural leveler except where age, educational level, poverty, or language may constitute a cultural barrier. Still, most of the young, a large number of adults, and a growing percentage of the older population are becoming accustomed to and grounded in using this and related technologies.

With thousands of Internet sites available related to health, questions of quality and veracity loom large. How many of these sites can be trusted? Some of the red flags that indicate a need for caution include those sites selling a product or service, vague information with no legitimate references, emotional testimonials, attacks on the medical establishment, and overzealous claims regarding the miraculous benefits and safety of a product. Education and caution become vital tools in successful health-related use of the Internet.

The consumer is not the only one using the Web for information. Health professionals and researchers are also benefiting from the Internet and electronic communications, and in ways that go beyond searching or managing ever-bourgeoning evidence and publication databases. New information technologies connect professionals, experts, and researchers, allowing them to network and share vital information.

The Internet is also becoming a primary tool in public health surveillance and early disease detection. Sources including government agencies, press reports, blogs, and chat rooms contribute to distribution

•

of public health information not only nationally, but globally. Brownstein, Freifeld, and Madoff report that "the advent of openly available news aggregators and visualization tools has spawned a new generation of disease-surveillance 'mashups' (Web application hybrids) that can mine, categorize, filter, and visualize online intelligence about epidemics in real time" (2008).

Although these new information technologies are extremely promising, they, too, are vulnerable to false reports, overload, media involvement, and security issues. They will require careful monitoring, verification, and evaluation.

TELEMEDICINE

Telemedicine concerns the incorporation and use of modern electronic communications systems to transmit medical information from one site to another, enabling care to be delivered from a distance. Transmission may be through videoconferencing, still images and data, and educational programs for medical personnel, facilitating administration and research. Medical records may also be stored and transferred through telemedical technology as these records become "digitized." Care can thus be offered to patients in isolated or underserved areas, including consultations with specialists when needed. The U.S. military is also researching telemedicine for delivery of care on the battlefield. A surgeon in one location, for example, may perform surgery using robotics to operate on patients in another location (Darkins and Cary 2000).

While telemedicine in various forms is available in all states and is expected to grow in usage and potential, the issues of privacy, security, adequate infrastructure, licensure and malpractice issues for out-of-state consultations, initial programs, and training all pose difficulties. Still, the potential for use in public health crises, natural disasters, or terrorist attacks is well recognized (Darkins and Cary 2000).

From a cultural perspective, it will be interesting to see who derives the most benefit from the spread of e-health communication technologies. With concomitant changes appearing in all parts of the health care system, including doctor-patient relationships, methods of caregiving, spread of previously guarded or unavailable information, treatment modalities, new discoveries and applications, growing patient diversity, and accompanying ethical dilemmas, the entire health care system is changing—this in spite of efforts to resist made by vested commercial interests and those who simply fear change.

ELECTRONIC MEDICAL RECORDS

Another innovative use of information technology is the move from paper to electronic medical records. Not only does this decrease paper waste and increase the transportability of medical records; it also helps with legibility as orders and so on are typed in.

Moreover, keeping records in electronic databases makes aggregate data use much easier than the past. This is important for tracking things such as, for instance, whether one drug is associated with better outcomes than another, or if, say, the use of certain diagnostic equipment actually serves to identify more actual cases of a given condition —or leads to more complications and unnecessarily raises costs. Data searches for individual patients, too, can be helpful.

The Veterans Health Administration has been a pioneer not only in the use of electronic medical records but also in creating systems to examine and tag patient records as needed with physician reminders (e.g., to conduct certain screening tests). Research indicates that computerized clinical reminders improve adherence to established clinical guidelines (Demakis et al. 2000; Morgan, Goodson, and Barnett 1998). Further, they can increase access to care: Patients who do not realize or are too stigmatized to explicitly say that they are at risk for certain conditions (e.g., HIV/AIDS) can be identified through routine medical record searches (see Sobo et al. 2008).

The promise of electronic records brings with it certain concerns, including possible threats to patient privacy and the potential misuse of patient data. There is also concern that computers in the examining room could come between doctor and patient; this, however, seems not to have been the case.

MEDICAL HOME

A number of new health care delivery models also are being explored. One such is the **Medical Home**. In contrast to the present model, whereby various services are fragmented with patients getting (immunizations from one location, acute care from another, specialist care from another, medications from another, and so forth), the medical home is patient centered. It seeks to strengthen doctor-patient relationships by coordinating patient care with a focus on an ongoing relationship through a team approach led by primary care physicians (see Fisher 2008).

This model focuses mainly on care coordination but, in the process, it also promises more personalized care, better use of community resources, and better patient outcomes. It could also reduce avoidable costs, improve quality of care, and include more patient involvement throughout the life cycle. This would facilitate preventive and chronic care.

Realistically, there are a number of barriers to the model, such as requirements for participation, payment reforms, full access to medical information and records by relevant medical personnel, physician collaboration, safety of sharing medical information through electronic means, and portability or transfer of care when patients move to other areas. The largest barrier may be referrals outside the medical home and the question of incentives when hospitals and specialists see the volume of patients fall with fewer visits, hospital stays, and diagnostic tests. According to Fisher, "The medical home has great potential to improve the provision of primary care and the financial stability of primary care practice. What has been missing so far has been an effort to implement this model in concert with other reforms that more effectively align the interests of all physicians and hospitals toward the improvement of patient care" (2008, 1202).

Another innovation adopted to address the need for coordinated hospital care has been the introduction of "hospitalists"—doctors that work for and in one hospital rather than as visiting nonemployees with permission to treat inpatients on the premises. Hospitalists have been described as if Mississippi river boat pilots, who guide larger boats through the river's treacherous currents, bring them to safety, and once there, hand over control once again to the ship's captain (Slataper 1997, 5–6). The hospitalist serves as the physician-of-record for inpatients who are accepted from primary care providers, cares for them during the hospital stay, and hands them back to their physician at discharge. Being present throughout the patient's hospital stay, the hospitalist can coordinate care and react to clinical data, relieving the primary physician of frequent hospital visits and keeping track of patient care. The primary physician also has fewer disruptions to his or her ambulatory or regular practice. It is true that occasional problems in communication and possible patient dissatisfaction from being assigned to an outside, unknown physician can arise (Wachter 1999). Still, in their review of the hospitalist movement, Bishop and Kathuria note: "The literature is clear that hospitalists lower costs and shorten the length of hospital admissions without diminishing the quality of patient care" (2008, 428).

The cultural relevance, however, of the hospitalist and other developments just outlined has not been addressed, and broad disparities remain. All people must first have access to the system, to benefit from innovations within the system. Delivery and financing must therefore form the context for innovations, quality, and equitable care.

REFORM AND THE SYSTEM

There is little argument that the American health care system has long been in need of reform. The United States is the only Western industrial nation that does not have some form of **universal health care** (basic care for all or a large majority of the population). The challenge is not only to make the system cost effective and to provide for the health care needs of all to the greatest extent possible, but to make the system more tolerant of and responsive to other cultural values and approaches, which is vital in the production of health and prevention and treatment of illness.

This would mean moving away from the biomedical model as the single acceptable approach, and toward a more integrated and inclusive model that considers the patient as a whole, multidimensional person, and affirms that healing is psychological, social, spiritual, and cultural, as well as biological. Such a shift would, in turn, entail some major structural changes in the face of not only biomedical but also corporate resistance, as well as the value structure and belief system of the U.S. population.

In 1981, Imershein cited both Navarro (1973; 1976) and Alford (1975) explaining the reasons for so little change in the face of what was already at that time a continuing crisis. Navarro, using a Marxist perspective, found the problem rooted in the fundamental economic structure of the society, while Alford related it to the distribution of power and control. From both perspectives, the possibilities for significant change would seem bleak to nil.

Imershein did note "a lot going on" (1981, 2). However, he proposed that even with all of the various experiments in corporate health maintenance organizations and government involvement in financing, establishment of regulatory health systems agencies, the expansion of training for physician assistants and allied paraprofessionals, and the emergence of a family practice specialty, that the system would basically absorb the changes, rather than undergoing significant change to address the underlying problems. That is what seems to have occurred. Costs continue to rise, and more people go without care. Poor minorities in this category now are being joined by some from middle class and professional sectors. Why has reforming the system been so difficult?

GENERAL RESISTANCE TO CHANGE

Change produces reactions, and the more radical the change, the more resistance may be generated. While change may be spurred by demand as well as by economic and social necessity, those who fear what is different or unknown and those who have vested interests in the status quo will tend to strongly resist and act to defeat any attempts at what they perceive as radical change (Schaefer 2000). National health insurance, for example, is frightening to many who are suspicious of and opposed to government involvement and control.

Vested interests include physicians who fear limits on income, private insurance companies that could be put out of business, and pharmaceutical companies that could lose profits if competitive pricing and legally imported drugs or research on and development of cheaper but effective alternative medicines and treatments were allowed and promoted. It would be in the interest of these entities, then, to resist any significant change they do not perceive of as to their benefit.

The use of the media is significant in thwarting any efforts to restructure the system. For example, in response to the Clinton Health Care Reform Plan, a television commercial was created by the advertising firm of Goddard Claussen and funded by the Health Insurance Association of America. It featured two white, middle-class individuals, Harry and Louise, seated at their dining room table, despairing over the bureaucratic nature of the plan, lamenting that they could not choose their own doctor with the slogan "let the government choose, we lose." It was immensely successful, and contributed a great deal to defeat of the plan—so much so that Harry and Louise were revived for the 2009 health care reform debates.

If a population is frightened of changes they do not understand or if they fear losing whatever they might have, they are vulnerable to many forms of propaganda and confusion. Common tactics include name-calling, framing an argument or an individual in negative or general terms that are essentially meaningless, or associating a person or policy with negative or positive images and slogans. "Just plain folks" or the middle class or "working families" are often invoked as victims or advocates. Most appeals give only one side of an issue or argument, neglecting any information opposed to the given position. There is often an attempt to make it appear that a majority is in favor of or opposed to an issue (Henslin 2007, 633).

Cultural factors also may shape the resistance to change. Historically based lack of trust in the majority's or the government's motives is frequently noted as contributing to resistance to various policy changes in some minority groups such as among Native Americans and African Americans (see Chapter 2).

In 1937, William Ogburn noted that resistance to change was often encouraged by the fact that the material culture (e.g., technology) changes much more rapidly than nonmaterial culture. Ogburn termed this **culture lag**. For example the use of imaging in medicine, and particularly the mapping of the human genome with all the implications for genetic medicine, may frighten or anger those whose religious beliefs may be in conflict. One such arena for such resistance is in regard to stem cell research.

Social change creates strain and uncertainty, and people may even take positions against their own best interests. The world, however, continues to change and will not remain static. Hopefully, we will learn to create nonmaterial cultural adaptations more quickly, or we will be unable to cope with the material changes occurring more and more rapidly throughout the world.

STAKEHOLDER RESISTANCE TO CHANGE

Many changes that take place within the system may be resisted by some or all of the various stakeholders affected by the new processes. For example, some doctors worry that the management-imposed use of clinical guidelines devalues the art of medicine. Veterans Health Administration providers in one study felt that their computerized clinical reminder system likewise disenfranchised them as professionals: as physicians who were able to recognize patient care needs by themselves, unassisted. Some also worried that the reminder system might be used for surveillance purposes, adding to performance pressures they already keenly felt. Nurses had their own reasons for resistance, some having to do with the power structure in the clinic. Information technologists resented the partial way that they were included in the reminder's design and deployment (Sobo et al. 2008, 219).

Health care organizations have acknowledged the challenge of implementing quality improvement interventions. Indeed, a new field, variously termed "implementation science," "translation research," and "quality improvement research," has emerged to address this. This development fits very well with the mainstream culture's valuation of audit and accountability practices as well as the growing sophistication with which even lay people are coming to understand that culture is everywhere—even in the clinic, where nurse culture, medical doctor culture, surgeon culture, management culture, clerk culture, patient culture, and so on often clash.

GLOBAL HEALTH CARE, GLOBALIZED HEALTH

To a certain degree, biomedicine's interest in culture was spurred by involvement in post-World War II international or global health initiatives. Organizations like the World Health Organization provided an institutional basis for expressing such interest, on foreign soil. But multiculturalism in health care has become a global issue in another way in the past decades, as populations increasingly (and with increasing speed, for example via jet airplane) travel to other countries as residents, refugees, or tourists. Diseases know no boundaries and travel with their hosts. Insects, viruses, and pollution do not require passports. Viruses that once may have fizzled out in place now may produce a worldwide pandemic, as in the spread of HIV/AIDS, and, more recently, drug-resistant tuberculosis, SARS (severe acute respiratory syndrome), and the H1N1 flu virus. Human activity is basically responsible for new global threats to health and well-being. Overuse of antibiotics (which produces drug-resistant disease strains), pollution of air, water, and food, global warming, poor sanitation, overcrowded populations of people, animals, and birds and their interactions, and international trade are taking their toll. Substance abuse, interpersonal violence, accidents and injuries, lack of health care facilities, and noncompliance or the inability to comply of patients who may receive only intermittent care all add to the problems.

However, global disparities in the distribution of wealth reinforce the fact that the poor and marginalized are hardest hit. Their populations, and especially their children, are more vulnerable to urban pollution, chemical, physical, and biological hazards. For example, more than 40 percent of the total disease burden (in terms of disability adjusted life years lost) due to air pollution occurs in developing countries (World Health Organization). Development strategies that do not aim to create safe environments in support of sustainable human health represent a step backward, not forward, for the global poor.

Global health problems do not concern only the developing world, as many might think. They affect every nation, directly and indirectly, economically, politically, and morally: "Health is the foundation for civil society, for social and cultural growth, for political stability, and for economic sustainability" (Global Health Initiative 2008). Illness and poverty create instability and unrest worldwide.

Solutions to global health problems require the interaction and cooperation of national governments and diverse health care systems. Research must be shared; epidemiological and other information tracked, recorded, and disseminated; and treatments coordinated and planned. Sharing and cooperation must be as blind to national boundaries as are the health problems being addressed. The Global Health Initiative notes that the United States can and must be a leader in addressing these problems with research, diagnostic tests, preventive measures, treatments, and vaccines due to their available resources and leadership. Products must be developed and distributed. Local sustainability plans must be created and implemented. Health care professionals in this country and abroad must be trained for practice under resource-poor conditions.

One force for multicultural change and the generation of appropriately trained (i.e., culturally sensitive) health care workers is the medical travel industry. In part due to "the liberalization of trade in services, the growing cooperation between private and public sectors, the easy global spread of information about products and services, and, most importantly, the successful splicing of the tourism and health sectors" (Bookman and Bookman 2007, 95), patients outbound from various North American and European nations have joined the medical travel consumer population. In the United States, thanks to (among other things) high numbers of uninsured and underinsured individuals, an increasing demand for so-called lifestyle care, such as aesthetic or cosmetic surgery, technological developments allowing for quicker, less invasive and cheaper surgical procedures, increased awareness of options due to word of mouth regarding the quality and value of outsourced care (including Internet discussions), and increased general media coverage of medical tourism, the number of medical travelers is growing at astounding rates. Estimates put the number of Americans traveling abroad for medical care in 2007 at 750,000; the anticipated number for 2010 is 6 million (Keckley and Underwood 2008, 3).

While some outbound travelers seek treatments unavailable at home, the majority of medical travel has been explained by financial logic: A hip replacement costs about $37,000 in the United States and about $13,000 in India. An $80,000 U.S. heart bypass is $16,000 in Thailand (Higgins, 2007). Using weighted average procedure prices, Deloitte put the average savings from the U.S. perspective at about 85 percent (Keckley and Underwood 2008). Moreover, care procured at certified facilities is generally of equal or better quality than the U.S. standard (Milstein and Smith 2006).

Medical travel will certainly be a fruitful arena for increasing our understanding of other cultures, and of culture contact. Too often we see the exchange of ideas and practices as a one-way transfer from the West. In actuality, the exchange flows both ways. For example, foreign-generated models of care can be adapted and incorporated domestically.

Beyond cultural artifacts and ideas, patients are traveling across borders, with ramifications for social arrangements and cultural practices. The concern here is not just foreign nationals such as U.S. citizens seeking offshore services, and their local impact. Of concern, too, are foreign or migrant workers who now may find it easier to return to their own countries for health care. Someone from India, say, who lives in the United States or England can more easily now than in generations past return home for cardiac or other necessary health care rather than undergoing procedures on foreign ground— and they can do so more safely, too, in terms of overall increases in the availability of high-quality care in many developing nations (Milstein and Smith 2006). Importantly, returning citizens may receive care that is more culturally relevant to them. Trips home may serve to reinvigorate or reconfigure kinship connections and ethnic identities, or stimulate the development of new cultural practices. Moreover, they may help bolster their nations' health care industries, adding to the synergies already building.

Like migrant patients, providers also can more easily return home, and so they too may help strengthen their homelands' health care offerings. Nations such as Trinidad and India have seen doctors return home to practice now that they can do so in world-class facilities (*Economist* 2008a). Nurses, doctors, and other health care specialists who previously emigrated to places like the United States may return home; many may stay home when practicing there becomes more practical. Their newly stationary careers will, of course, affect the flow of ideas and practices. In addition to benefiting their homeland, the decrease in numbers of providers willing to travel to the United States may affect, quite significantly, the makeup of our own health care workforce labor supply.

But overseas, jobs may be created: Hospitals—even those catering to medical travelers—employ local residents. Job creation may even lead more residents in medical travel supply zones to seek out medical training, adding to local knowledge and perhaps increasing the sustainability of programs serving the local poor as well, some of whom may find employment in hospitals. The policy climate is clearly important here, not only in terms of workforce issues but also in terms of policies meant to ensure that a portion of medical travel profits themselves are earmarked for the poor, and that the poor are not exploited by the industry.

Exploitation may happen, for instance, in response to the globalized demand for transplant organs or gestational surrogates. The latter, for example, may exploit poor women, putting them at risk for complications during surgical impregnation, gestation, and childbirth (for instance when cesarean sections are called for, to time the birth as desired by the legal parents) and it discourages adoption and fostering.

However, the poor were neglected or maltreated by many nations' health care systems long before the medical travel industry coalesced (*Economist* 2008b). And competition introduced from outside of the United States may in fact stimulate improvement in health care offerings in these nations. Time will tell.

The exigencies of addressing health care on a global scale add additional force to the need for reform. In addition, the implications for cultural diversity and multicultural understanding are huge, since training personnel, meeting and cooperating internationally, and developing strategies for treatment and prevention that are culturally consistent and relevant all require a multicultural approach. As the globe becomes smaller, we must learn from each other to benefit the whole.

THE NEED FOR A MULTICULTURAL ORIENTATION

For some people, both within and outside of the health care professions, the idea of the need for cultural understanding and sensitivity in health care is still a controversial issue. However, from a practical and professional perspective, the practice of medicine is best understood as naturally multicultural. Where the culture of biomedicine comes into contact with other medicines and other cultures, it is also syncretic. Each may borrow and learn from the other, incorporating and adapting techniques and philosophies. This requires communication and mutual respect.

Biomedicine, as a service-oriented profession dedicated to the alleviation of suffering for people of all cultures, has a responsibility to reexamine its own motivations, goals, and ethical ideals. Cure must be reconciled with care, and care must be conceptualized in ways consistent with patient perceptions. In the next chapter, we discuss a number of ways that medical care providers can become more culturally sensitive in order to enhance both their curing and their caring.

FOR DISCUSSION

1. What are some cultural aspects of bioethics, from both patient and provider viewpoints?

2. Why has reform of the health care system been so difficult to achieve? What are the major barriers? How might these barriers be overcome?

3. What are the major issues that may arise when new information technologies are introduced into health care? How are new technologies affecting the biomedical model?

4. Discuss the global aspects of health care today and how they affect the delivery of health care across national borders as well as within countries?

5. Can the orientations of profit and public service be compatible?

CHAPTER 7
Developing Cultural Sensitivity

GOAL: Comprehend the possible dangers of assuming that even when the same language is spoken, communication between patient and practitioner is nonproblematic; understand the range of potential barriers to verbal and nonverbal communication.

GOAL: Define cultural sensitivity (also called cultural competence) and describe processes entailed in its implementation, including basic activities necessary for learning about the patient perspective.

GOAL: Examine socialization and motives of health care professionals to illuminate how patients can more productively interact with them.

When we think of all [the] tasks in the consultation, what is surprising is not how often we fail, but that we ever succeed. Even when patients and doctors come from a common culture, neither participant has any idea what the other is talking about much of the time. In one sense, every consultation can be thought of as a cross-cultural one.

(Fuller and Toon 1988, 27–28)

Because of the disease orientation of biomedicine and the tendency to medicalize or reduce problems to the organic level, recommendations for diagnosis and treatment within the biomedical system did not, until recently, begin to include the consideration of cultural beliefs, values, or practices. The great impact these have on health and illness has long been demonstrated by social scientists. Increasingly, MDs are getting social science PhDs too—and sharing social science insights within the biomedical community (e.g., Farmer 1999, 2005; Helman 2007; Kleinman 1980; Waitzkin 2001). Culture can no longer be ignored by biomedical professionals.

While the nursing profession has for some time promoted the benefits of "culture care" (Leininger 1985), many physicians may still resist the suggestion that they should address a patient's emotional and psychological needs as well as his or her physiological problems, and they may not see the benefits of doing so. As one physician asked Loustaunau, "Do you mean to tell me that when I'm trying to treat a patient or save a life, I should be considering their cultural values and attitudes? That is utterly absurd!"

This viewpoint reflects the reductionist model of medical care, excluding the role of social and psychological factors in health and illness. It is true that being culturally sensitive can entail a great deal of extra study, effort, and time. But considering the multicultural nature of the U.S. population, and demographic projections for increasing multiculturalization, cultural sensitivity is a key prerequisite for effective treatment.

In 2001, the U.S. government issued national standards for culturally and linguistically appropriate services (CLAS) in health care, and these included mandates for all recipients of federal funds as well as guidelines and recommendations. The mandates, based on Title VI of the Civil Rights Act of 1964, include directives to provide language assistance services, including bilingual staff and interpreters as well as signage and printed matter in languages common to groups in the service area.

The accompanying guidelines and recommendations begin with the statement that "health care organizations should ensure that patients/consumers receive from all staff members effective, understandable, and respectful care that is provided in a manner compatible with their cultural health beliefs and practices and preferred language." It is suggested that mandated linguistic services should be part of a larger effort aimed at the provision of culturally sensitive care more generally.

Commonly termed **cultural competence**, the approach is defined officially as "a set of congruent behaviors, attitudes, and policies that come together in a system, agency, or among professionals that *enables effective work in cross-cultural situations*" (Office of Minority Health, 2005, emphasis ours). As Brach and Fraser observe: "Cultural competency is an explicit statement that one-size-fits-all health care cannot meet the needs of an increasingly diverse American population" (2000, 183). Care that is sensitive to cultural background is required. Although more research is needed on actual medical outcomes for patients who receive culturally sensitive care and patients who do not, the research that has been done suggests that culturally sensitive care can affect patient compliance or adherence to a given care plan as well as patient satisfaction, comfort, and attitude toward the medical establishment.

Organizational imperatives notwithstanding, such as the need for a more diverse workforce as well as for operational processes that reflect and support the tenets of cultural competence, for practitioners an awareness that the perceptions patients hold may differ from biomedical ones, and that patients need to be made to feel comfortable if they are to discuss their concerns, is key. Developing the ability to communicate is, therefore, essential (Sobo and Seid 2003). Another strategy for clinicians who would be culturally sensitive is to develop networks of contacts within the communities to be served. And most important of all, they need to develop sensitivity to health needs as defined by those communities. As Fuller and Toon have noted, "The greater the cultural distance between doctor and patient, the less likely their expectations of the consultation and its outcome are to be congruent" (1988, 27; see also Cockerham 2010, Chapter 9; Philipsen 2003).

ISSUES OF COMMUNICATION

THE PROBLEM OF COMPLIANCE

Doctors often become frustrated when patients do not comply with instructions, and it is estimated that over 60 percent of patients who visit biomedical practitioners are to some degree noncompliant (DiMatteo and DiNicola 1982; also see Cameron 1996). The reasons for this are varied, but the rejection of or failure to act on instructions is generally not due to a patient's unncooperative nature or ignorance, as some doctors conclude.

For example, Snow tells of a young first-time mother whose baby was failing to gain weight. After numerous consultations and one hospitalization, the pediatrician recommended a special formula high in calories and nutrients. The mother began to cry. As Snow explains, "A few questions revealed that she had not had enough money to buy formula in the first place and, when told that her baby needed a certain number of ounces/day, she had diluted the bottles to make sure that he got the proper amount" (1993, 245). Current research continues to reveal similar findings.

However, financial stress is not the only cause for noncompliance; if it were, we would expect to find total compliance among those with financial resources, when we do not (Cameron 1996). This is because factors other than money, such as cultural expectations for consultations or for medication's effects, can influence care plan adherence. Information we have on this subject is limited mostly to biomedical consultations. Whether people comply more, or less, and why, to nonbiomedical practitioner recommendations definitely needs further investigation, as does the problem of patient reticence to share compliance (and other) information with providers.

Much of this sharing problem has to do with people's aversion to the possibility of being judged as inferior by providers who do not share their cultural background, or of being lectured by providers who do not understand the constraints of poverty—or of religious rules regarding certain medical practices, and so on (e.g., Prussing et al. 2004; Prussing et al. 2005; Sobo, Seid, and Gelhard 2006). But other factors also are at work. Many patients have unrealistic expectations for providers' intuitive ability to discern their problems, to determine exactly what they need, and for what medicine can reasonably accomplish. These perceptions have been encouraged by the idea that physicians are, or should be, infallible and all-seeing. The media has also encouraged the idea that there is a pill for everything, and that anything can be "fixed."

Because the term "compliance" implies a power differential between practitioner and patient, as the relationship changes, the enhancement of compliance requires mutual trust and cooperation in decision making and implementation of treatment. The remedy should then lie in the communication process.

COMPLIANCE AND INTERCULTURAL COMMUNICATION

A reasonable amount of time is necessary for good communication to take place but communication also requires a number of skills: One must be able to express oneself in a manner understood by others and one must be able to listen to and properly interpret information offered and questions asked by others. Previous knowledge and experience can affect the efficacy of both expression and interpretation in both physician and patient.

One of the measures of communication is how much information gets transmitted. The need for information rather than treatment may actually be what brings many patients to clinicians. Some people go only for a diagnosis. Further, some go only for ailments that are new to them. Others go to make sure a condition is under control or to confirm their own treatment regimen is working (see Cockerham 2010, 134–56; Snow 1993, 129).

However much patients may desire information, findings from studies cited in Hahn's 1995 review of the literature on patient-practitioner interaction suggests that one in five patients ask no questions at all and that 13 percent of patient questions go unanswered (169). Patients in one study of biomedical consultations spent an average of only eight seconds asking questions. Physicians in the study believed that they spent an average of nine full minutes providing information when in actuality they spent an average of 1.3 minutes doing so (Waitzkin 1985, 89). Compliance based on maybe 80 seconds worth of information transmission may, by definition, be problematic—especially when patient recall of doctor's explanations and instructions has been reported at only 50 percent (Hahn 1995, 168).

Work done more recently has helped to flesh out the picture developed in the 1980s. As noted in Kessells's 2003 review, "40–80% of medical information provided by healthcare practitioners is forgotten immediately. The greater the amount of information presented, the lower the proportion correctly recalled; furthermore, almost half of the information that is remembered is incorrect" (219). Recall will vary by condition, education level, linguistic issues, and so on. It also will vary by provider or educator characteristics, such as time spent with patient, completeness of information provided, whether or not visual aids were used, and the like.

The power structure of many biomedical consultations compounds the problem by limiting the role of the patient. So do class differences: Waitzkin identified a class-based cultural communication barrier (1985, 98). American working-class patients may tend to communicate more with tone and gesture than directly. Physicians, who are mainly from middle- and upper-class backgrounds, may be accustomed to direct verbal inquiries and so may fail to hear the nonverbal questions.

Further, even people who speak the same language or share the same language base can "talk past" each other. Cultural rules, including rules regarding doctor-patient consultations, are generally implicit or tacit and "each party assumes without discussion that it is their rules that both are using" (Fuller and Toon 1988, 28), even when they are not.

The language of the biomedical culture is grounded in bodies and their mechanics, diagnoses, and repair. But the medical lexicon also serves to bind the medical community together and helps its members express the reality of their own lives and experiences; it also distinguishes them from nonmedical personnel and patients. Notwithstanding, the use in clinics of the biomedical slang referred to as "medspeak" or "doc talk" and the rationalization by clinicians that communication is not important because patients could not possibly understand medical terminology adds to the communication gap.

Patients also have their own culturally related lexicons. And even when they do have some familiarity with biomedical terminology, whether slang or technical jargon, miscommunication may occur. Patients and clinicians may use medical terminology in different ways. For example, people who report having "high blood," "pressure," or "high-pertension" do not refer to the same things that clinicians do when they say "hypertension" or "high blood pressure." First, while the last two terms are the same to clinicians, for certain black people "high-pertension" means increased tension or stress, combined with increased blood volume. Pressure, or "high blood," on the other hand, just means having too much blood, or blood that is therefore too high in the body (Heurtin-Roberts and Reisin 1990; Snow 1993, 117–34).

Hypertension, biomedically defined, is something altogether different, so it is important to make sure that when similar terms are used that the meanings attributed also are the same. If not, adherence to clinician suggestions will likely be poor, as the physician will not address the problem that really concerns the patient.

MEDICAL INTERPRETATION AND TRANSLATION

People who do not speak the same primary or native language have an even more difficult time communicating in the clinic setting. The most obvious strategy when provider and patient do not speak the same language is to use an interpreter (an interpreter conveys meaning orally; a translator conveys meaning in writing). But, as demonstrated in early studies on the subject, simply finding someone who speaks the same language as the patient is not enough.

For example, it is important that written material be translated for the patient or his or her family, as advice might not be fully remembered after a consultation (and it should not be assumed that people always can read the languages that they speak). It also is essential that instructions given (e.g., how to cleanse a healing wound at home) are given in logical sequence; if x precedes y, then instructions should be stated that way: "Do x and then y" (e.g., Fuller and Toon 1988, 46). Asking the recipient of instructions to repeat them back helps to confirm their comprehension.

The interpreter must be perceived of as nonthreatening and encouraging to the patient (Fuller and Toon 1988, 45; Tseng and Streltzer 2008, 31–32). Moreover, the interpreter must interpret the clinician's communications exactly, without editing or altering what is said. This means that idiomatic expressions, which may not make sense when translated literally into another language, must be converted so that their meanings remain intact in the target language. We are reminded of a friend who had a visitor from another country to dinner. Having eaten his fill, the man announced that he was "fed up." Had the hosts not known about the man's culture, they may have interpreted what he said as aggressive and insulting.

Two more examples help illustrate the problematic nature of idiomatic expressions. Both are taken from Geri-Ann Galanti's U.S. case study collections (1991, 2008), as are most of the other examples used in this section. The first example involves a mistakenly literal translation of "cold feet" or apprehension so that a Chinese-born physician suspected circulatory disease. In a different but similar case, a Korean physician who sought to reassure a patient when the patient nervously but jokingly asked if he would "kick the bucket" answered very positively, but to the wrong effect, " 'Oh, yes, you are definitely going to kick the bucket!' " (2008, 27).

These examples are doubly significant. Not only do they demonstrate how nonsensical idiomatic expressions can be, but they also show that the linguistically divergent individual need not be the patient. And they show, also, that interpretation may be happening in an individual's own thoughts and not just through a trained interpreter or translator.

Some health care settings have paid interpreters and translators on call who provide professional and continuous service, resulting in a patient–interpreter/translator–clinician team that persists for the duration of the treatment. Such continuity is very important. Some clinics even have cross-cultural advocates or brokers: "trained members of a particular ethnic group who act as go-betweens for that group and the institution" (Fuller and Toon 1988, 37). Advocates interpret but also educate health workers about their cultures and the economic and health problems typical among members of their group. They review health education materials that target their group; assist patients in understanding their options, for example, as in regard to surgery and its implications; and help staff members understand, and thereby reduce, institutional racism (37).

Many clinics and hospitals cannot afford this service, let alone professional interpreters or translators, despite the government's (unfunded) mandate for them, as per the CLAS standards (described earlier). If a member of staff speaks a language common to the patient population, he or she might be called upon. A friend or relative of a patient might also serve as an interpreter in an emergency.

Despite their best intentions, relatives who volunteer do not always provide good translations or interpretations. Besides their lack of familiarity with medical terms and procedures, they have other roles to play in relation to the patient, and certain role expectations may conflict with the messages they are asked to relay by clinicians. Moreover, clinicians must think carefully about patients' right to confidentiality, which should not be violated; patients may not wish to reveal certain details in the presence of family or friends.

For example, a woman accompanied by a husband or boyfriend may not want him to know about past abortions, sexually transmitted diseases, contraceptive use, or pregnancies. Her concerns about self-presentation and preserving her self-esteem and that of others may override her interest in meeting the clinician's need for accuracy. Talk of reproductive matters between children and parents also can be problematic, as the following example shows:

A Hispanic woman, Graciela Mendoza, had to sign an informed consent form for a hysterectomy. Her bilingual son served as the interpreter. When he described the procedure to his mother, he appeared to be translating accurately and indicating the appropriate body parts. His mother signed willingly. The next day, however, when she learned that her uterus had been removed and that she could no longer bear children, she became very angry and threatened to sue the hospital. What went wrong?

Because it is inappropriate for a Hispanic male to discuss the private parts of his mother, the embarrassed son explained that a tumor would be removed from her abdomen and pointed to that general area. When Mrs. Mendoza learned that her uterus had been removed, she was quite angry and upset because a Hispanic woman's status is derived in large part from the number of children she produces.

(Galanti 2008, 39)

As Galanti has noted, "Even speaking the same language is not always sufficient. Cultural rules often dictate who can discuss what with whom" (1991, 16). Another important aspect of this case is the way in which the translator edited for the mother. Editing also can happen in the other direction: Some translators will consider themselves representatives of their culture or of the person for whom they are translating, and they will take pains to eliminate any statement that might reflect poorly on the patient or on their group.

NONVERBAL COMMUNICATION

EXPRESSIVITY

Cultural rules dictate who talks about what, to whom, and also when discussion should take place to begin with, as well as at what pace it should proceed at and at what decibel (Kreps and Kunimoto 1994, 116). Members of some cultures tend to be loud and verbally expressive when they wish to demonstrates interest and concern.

Silence is another form of expression, and its value is quite high in some cultures. This can have ramifications for provider-patient interaction:

Ellen was trying to teach her Navaho patient, Jim Nez, how to live with his newly diagnosed diabetes. She soon became extremely frustrated because she felt she was not getting through to him. He asked very few questions and never met her eyes. She reasoned from this that he was uninterested and therefore not listening to her.

Rather than signaling disinterest, however, Mr. Nez's behavior demonstrated a respect for the nurse's authority. The Navaho value silence. A person who interrupts while someone is speaking is perceived as immature. Most Americans are uncomfortable with silences and tend to fill them with words, making "small" talk. The Navaho use silence to formulate their thoughts. Words should have significance.

(Galanti 1991, 16)

Silence may signal respect, but again, it may not: It may reflect fear. A Laotian refugee being treated for stomach cancer refused to talk to a hospital social worker because, says Galanti, she seemed to "have feared that anything she said would have repercussions for her family still in Laos and Thailand" (1991, 28). Silence also may signal embarrassment at a lack of command of one's host country's language. In traditional Chinese and Japanese cultures, silence on the part of the speaker signals the listener to consider carefully the content of what was said before anyone goes on speaking. A black person may remain silent after being asked a question perceived as ridiculous. French, Spanish, and Russian people may interpret silence as signaling agreement (Fuller and Toon 1988, 4). Clearly, cultural context and individual acculturation levels must be taken into account when interpreting a silent reaction.

EXPRESSING PAIN

Pain is one of the symptoms used by biomedical practitioners in diagnosing illness; it is perceived as a signal that something is wrong. However, classic studies by Zborowski (1952) and Zola (1966) found that cultural ideas about expressiveness and stoicism influenced the expression of pain responses for several ethnic groups. Although this knowledge is important, with it as with other generalizations presented in this chapter and elsewhere, there is a consequent danger of inadvertent stereotyping and false expectations in physicians who treat these patients. Numerous other variables may intervene, such as age of patient, educational background, and personal experience. Still, such research shows that, to a significant degree, people may be willing to tolerate pain as a function of cultural expectations, sometimes even refusing medication.

One such case is described by Galanti. A Nigerian farmer was in the United States for surgery on a knee injury: "His nurse waited for him to request pain medication, but he never did. Mr. Seisay was Muslim, and he offered his pain to Allah in thanks for the good fortune of being allowed such specialized surgery" (Galanti 2008, 56).

Another case demonstrated how clinicians trained in one culture may easily misinterpret pain expressed in another:

[Mary Carroll] was scheduled for surgery at the end of the week. Her family became very concerned when she suddenly started complaining of pain. They knew Mrs. Carroll was typically Irish in her stoicism. They spoke to her doctor, who was from India. He was not worried. In his country, women were usually vocal when in pain. He ignored their requests that the surgery be done sooner, thinking it unnecessary.

When he finally did operate, he discovered that Mrs. Carroll's condition had progressed to the point that she could not be saved.

(Galanti 2008, 53–54)

These examples make clear how important it is for medical staff to be culturally aware of the relativity of the expression of pain.

OTHER MODES OF COMMUNICATION

Eye contact is another mode of communication that can have wide cultural variation. Patients may read a physician's gaze as reflecting knowledge and caring, which can inspire trust and reassurance—but not always. The patient gaze may also be misinterpreted. Aversion of the eyes can signal respect, as in the case of many Asian and West African cultures: "An English doctor with a West African patient may therefore feel that she or he is depressed, hostile, or not being straightforward, when in fact there is merely a difference of cultural convention. Conversely, the African patient may experience the English doctor's eye contact as excessive staring" (Fuller and Toon 1988, 51).

Sometimes, eyes are seen as spiritual windows, and so direct eye contact can endanger those involved. Other times, direct contact signals intimacy. Eye contact with certain patients might be misinterpreted as sexual interest; this can be distressing for all involved (Galanti 2008, 46).

Other forms of nonverbal communication that might become important during a consultation include one's physical proximity to patients. For instance, while many Americans, Canadians, and British people require substantial space between themselves and other people (Gross 1992, 109 reports this at about four feet), Latin American, Japanese, and Arabs prefer very little (about two feet for Latin Americans, according to Gross—who also cautions that most evidence on distance is anecdotal; and see Bente et al. 2008 regarding methodological problems in cross-cultural research on nonverbal behavior overall). Patients may attempt to pull clinicians into—or push them out of—personal space in order to make themselves more comfortable.

Habitual gestures also must be taken into account; they might have different meanings cross-culturally. While a nod of the head means "yes" to most Americans, Greek and some other Mediterranean people traditionally say "no" by a similarly vertical movement of the head (Gross 1992, 109). An American clinician might beckon a patient forward by wiggling the index finger out and in with the palm up and other fingers and thumb closed or bent in toward the palm. But this gesture is used in the Philippines to call animals (Galanti 1991, 22). Information on gestures relevant to the population(s) served by a clinic can help to avoid embarrassment.

COURTESY AND CIVILITY

Courtesy and civility can do much to enhance a relationship and improve communication. However, this form of expression too may be culturally relative. For example, some people may not wish to bother nurses, even when in pain, for to do so would be disrespectful.

A sense of politeness also might lead patients to answer "yes" when they really mean "no" or "maybe." For example, "rather than refuse to the physician's face and cause him dishonor" (1991, 21), a Chinese woman described by Galanti told her physician that she would return for follow-up treatment and then never did. Here is another example of this kind of situation:

Jackie, an Anglo nurse, was explaining the harmful side effects of the medication Adela Samillan, a Filipino patient, was to take at home after her discharge. Although Mrs. Samillan spoke some English, her husband who was more fluent, served as interpreter. Throughout Jackie's explanation, the Samillans nodded in agreement and understanding and laughed nervously. When Jackie verbally tested them on the information, however, it was apparent that they understood very little. What had happened?

Dignity and self-esteem are extremely important for most Asians. Had the Samillans indicated that they did not understand Jackie's instructions, they would have lost their self-esteem for not understanding or they would have caused Jackie to lose hers for not explaining the material well enough. By pretending to understand, Mr. and Mrs. Samillan felt they were preserving everyone's dignity.

(Galanti 2008, 30–31)

SHAME

One of the quickest ways to injure patient dignity is to write off their statements as old-fashioned or superstitious. When a Mexican-American mother says that her infant has *caída de mollera*, one group of physicians "would tell the mother not to believe in that kind of 'superstitious nonsense' " (Robert Trotter, as quoted in Arellano and Kearny 1992, 49). We hear this kind of comment today still, even though this is not an effective strategy.

Caída de mollera, or mollera caída, is a condition in which, among other things, an infant's anterior fontanel (the soft spot on the front of a baby's skull) is visibly depressed or has sunken or fallen in; the condition also is called "fallen fontanel." Other symptoms include excessive crying, reduced appetite, diarrhea, vomiting, restlessness, and irritability. The condition can be fatal without timely proper treatment; Trotter believes it is what biomedical specialists would call "severe dehydration." But because the women in Trotter's research knew that the clinicians would ridicule them, they would not bring the condition to the clinician's attention until it was very severe (as cited in Arellano and Kearny 1992, 49–50). Likewise, many do not tell clinicians about home remedies or complementary or alternative medical treatments they may be using (see Chapters 4 and 5).

Patients' use of their own terms should not be denigrated but rather encouraged if clinicians are to provide adequate care; a patient's use of the term caída de mollera can serve as a "good screening device" and a "significant indicator" that a child needs immediate attention (Arellano and Kearny 1992, 50). But how can clinicians find out about illnesses such as caída de mollera, let alone learn the terms for such illnesses, if patients are made to feel ashamed of them and then keep quiet?

The idea of becoming culturally sensitive may seem overwhelming in the face of all the possibilities. However, some common ethnographic methods can be incorporated into medical training, and adapted and utilized by health care professionals to enhance relationships and care, as well as to complement medical science with medical art. Ultimately, even mistakes will be much less serious if there is an open, trusting, and mutually respectful relationship between practitioner and patient.

ETHNOGRAPHIC TECHNIQUES: AN INTRODUCTION

Cultural sensitivity to communication practices, such as the ways in which the body is used or the people with whom it is appropriate to speak, is a first step in building sensitivity to other realms of culture as part of a culturally competent approach to the provision of health care. It is the first step in collecting and assessing further cultural data on a given aspect of a given way of life.

In order to enhance and facilitate communication, clinicians can try to gain an understanding of the particular cultural factors, which include ethnicity, sex, age, and social class, profession, and the like, to which different patient populations they serve subscribe—an ethnographic understanding. Technically, **ethnographies** are written accounts (-graphy) about certain peoples (ethno-). Libraries are full of such accounts, and this literature can be extremely helpful in familiarizing oneself with the culture of a patient population.

In addition to library resources, original research can also be useful and rewarding. A growing number of clinicians are joining or forming study groups specifically interested in doing research on the populations they serve. There are also a growing number of resources and manuals directed to health care providers that summarize and give general information on techniques of rapid assessment (e.g., Fuller and Toon 1988; Kreps and Kunimoto 1994; Tseng and Streltzer 2008; Srivastava 2007; Ring et al. 2008). Bernard (1995, 2001) provides a full discussion of the methods professional ethnographers might use, as do Pelto and Pelto (1996). Sobo (2009a) focuses specifically on ethnographic approaches in regard to today's health care challenges.

THE ETHNOGRAPHIC ASSESSMENT

While clinicians generally will not conduct full-fledged ethnographic research, they can collect ethnographic information by listening to what patients say about their lives. To gain insight into local social structures, clinicians should pay attention to the household forms most often described by patients. They also should attend to the types of individuals most often referred to by patients as emotional, social, and financial supports, and those most often cited as barriers, troublemakers, power brokers, or purse-string tighteners. Sometimes, in addition to individuals filling certain roles, such as father or cousin, specific community members occupying particular positions or offices will be named. The benevolence of those named community heroes may prove important if one wishes to gain the trust of the community.

One way clinicians can easily begin to collect social and cultural information is by getting out into the community and experiencing neighborhood life firsthand. This can be done, for example, by eating lunch in a local park or restaurant rather than in the office. The interested clinician can ask a fellow worker or a longtime patient who lives in or otherwise knows the area to accompany or guide her or him. Not only can this insider help to ease the clinician's entry, but his or her presence also might ensure the clinician's credibility.

Another way to increase awareness about the community being served is by paying attention to the media sources used by most members. Clinicians should find out what radio stations, newspapers, magazines, and TV shows or stations clinic users listen to, read, and watch. Clinicians can ask patients directly; short discussions about the media may be good for increasing patients' comfort level in the service site as well as for assisting clinicians in building a community profile. Clinicians can use what they learn not only for their own erudition, but also to ensure that their waiting rooms are stocked with reading material that patients find pertinent. We are reminded of a participant in Sobo's AIDS research (1997) who remarked that the waiting room of the agency supposed to be serving HIV-positive gay men had no gay newspapers or magazines. Unfortunately, this suggested to the man that he was not welcome there.

PARTICIPANT OBSERVATION

The main ethnographic method traditionally has been **participant observation**, in which the fieldworker participates as fully as possible in the life of the community while observing all that goes on. For example, an ethnographer interested in a healing church may help the pastor prepare for services as well as attending and participating in them, all the while recording incidents or data of interest. For instance, an ethnographer might record stories and songs, photograph tools used in healing services, and collect botanical samples or other medicinal substances deployed. An ethnographer interested in finding out more about what it is like to belong to a certain community will participate in and observe that community; he or she will make social contacts within that community, shop at local shops, attend local community meetings, and so on. Nonparticipant observation can also be done through simply observing and recording local happenings without any notable participation in what is being observed. Either way, one's full focus must be given; concentration skills necessary for this can be developed over time, with practice.

KEY INFORMANTS

As part of the participant observation process, but also as a stand-alone method, one can also build a network of people traditionally called **key informants**. Key or "good informants are people to whom you can talk easily, who understand the information you need, and who are glad to give it to you or get it for you" (Bernard 1995, 166). Key informants generally have the ability to intellectualize their culture and, if apprised of the theories that the researcher is formulating, will be able to tell the researcher if he or she is on the right track.

Key informants are strategically chosen; they are selected for their specialized knowledge. As Bernard notes, "In any given domain of culture, some people are more competent than others" (1995, 171). This makes the process of sampling, in which people are selected for their representativeness of the population in question, unnecessary for this kind of ethnographic inquiry.

For example, if one wished to find out about medicinal plants and their uses, the best person to ask would be an expert in that area. This would be much more efficient in terms of both time and effort than asking people randomly to tell you what they know about that cultural domain.

INTERVIEWS

One may gather culturally relevant data from key informants and other informants or, rather, **participants**—people willing to help with and participate in the research but not so intensively—through **ethnographic interviews**. Single interviews can be helpful, but repeated interviews carried out over time with the same individuals generally generate more valid and reliable information as trust accrues.

Participant observation entails constant **informal interviews**—casual, unplanned conversations in which important cultural facts are conveyed. For clinicians, however, much useful information can be collected through **formal interviews** during the clinical consultation. Formal interviews, like clinical interviews, involve purposefully sitting down with an informant to talk about a given topic. Yet, formal interviews need not be highly structured or controlled by the interviewer.

An **unstructured interview** would generally be conducted during the early stages of clinical contact as a way of simply warming people up to the idea of one's interest in their culture, and as a way of determining what kinds of questions structured interviews should entail. Bernard suggests, "Tell everyone you interview that you are trying to learn from *them*. Encourage them to interrupt you during the interview with anything they think is important" (1995, 211; emphasis in original). Let patient or participant concerns guide the flow of discussion. The ethnographer-clinician's greatest skill is to *listen*—a skill that should already be a part of the clinician's role and repertoire.

The emergent concerns of the participant should override predetermined questions at any time if the questions prove to be irrelevant, misguided, or culturally biased. A culturally biased question is one that forces a participant to think about an issue that he or she would not otherwise consider. People generally can come up with an answer, but if that answer never comes into play in real life, it is of little use to the clinician. Patients who are asked culturally biased questions also often tend to respond with what they think the inquirer wants to hear (cf. Bernard 1995, 231).

Culturally biased questions include those in which the categories used are those of the interviewer, not the interviewee. For example, Sobo (1996b) has demonstrated how abortion, as defined from a biomedical (etic) standpoint, may not be perceived as such by those being queried; Jamaicans, for example, like many other peoples, do not consider extracting a late menstrual period (menstrual regulation) as abortion. There are many reasons for this, one being that a fetus is not seen as a humanized potential baby until it becomes perceptibly active in the womb, which happens well after conception.

This example demonstrates how essential it is to find out how informants define terms or categories from their point of view before naively using categories in assessments. In the unstructured interview, a number of probing techniques are used to elicit such emic information. These include the **silent probe**, which Bernard defines as "just remaining quiet and waiting for an informant to continue" (1995, 215), sometimes with a nod or a mumbled "uh-huh." A **positive probe** involves an overtly stated "yes" or "I see." An **echo probe** encourages a participant to continue by echoing the last word or phrase said, in a questioning tone. ("Questioning tone?") Yes, the questioning tone provokes further elaboration. Another way to provoke talk is to construct a question such that extensive information is needed to respond to it, such as, "Tell me all the things you might do to stop diarrhea in your baby."

While the breadth of information that can be collected this way with unstructured interviewing, and the patient-driven nature of that information is invaluable, time constraints can make it impractical. Numerous heuristics and tools have been invented to save clinicians time and streamline the clinical interview process, with perhaps the most famous being eight brief questions sometimes referred to as "Kleinman's Questions" (Kleinman, Eisenberg, and Good 1978). These are:

1. What do you think caused your problem?
2. Why do you think it started when it did?
3. What do you think your sickness does to you?
4. How severe is your sickness? Do you think it will last a long time, or will it be better soon in your opinion?
5. What are the chief problems your sickness has caused for you?
6. What do you fear most about your sickness?
7. What kind of treatment would you like to have?
8. What are the most important results you hope to get from treatment?

Asking such questions can yield important information regarding the patient's "explanatory model" for what the problem is and how to fix it. Such information provides important support for arriving at an agreement regarding the best possible (most feasible, most culturally compatible) care plan.

In addition to specific questions that can be asked, a number of snappily-named heuristics have been invented to remind providers to practice cultural sensitivity. As Like notes in a recent editorial on the ongoing transformation of clinical practices to meet the nation's cross-cultural needs, we have tools such as "LEARN (Listen, Explain, Acknowledge, Recommend, Negotiate), BATHE (Background, Affect, Trouble, Handling, Empathy), ETHNIC (Explain, Treatment,

Healers, Negotiation, Intervention, Collaboration), and ESFT (Explanatory model, Social risks, Fears about medication, understanding Treatment)" (2005, 2189). Like provides, in the editorial, not only full references for these models but for the many helpful Web sites now existing to further the goal of culturally sensitive caring.

QUESTIONNAIRES

One of the main points of ethnography is to collect data concerning the issues as participants see them. This can be done with more structured, as well as less structured, methods. **Structured** data collection methods are used "to control the input that triggers each informant's responses so that the output can be reliably compared" (Bernard 1995, 237). Questionnaires, for example, fit this bill.

Using a questionnaire is a way of conducting **survey research**, or research in which a large number of people, and generally a carefully selected sample of them, are polled. **Questionnaires** generally consist of a page or more of questions that participants are asked to answer. They can be administered in person, by mail, over the phone, or in a variety of other ways. Brief questionnaires might be included with the required paperwork patients fill out on arriving for appointments.

The questions on questionnaires can be closed or open-ended. **Closed**, or forced-choice, questions force the participant to choose between two or more options. Sometimes the answers are provided in scale form (e.g., never, rarely, sometimes, often, always). **Open-ended** questions are those that respondents can answer as they like. The major themes that emerge in these answers can be identified after reading through them. Further, a theme coding scheme may be generated so that, as with closed-answer questionnaires, data collected can be quantified for processing.

One of the main problems in questionnaire construction is any given question's inherent ambiguity, so that each respondent answers what is, in the end, a different set of questions, making the results less useful than they might be. This has been made clear in HIV and AIDS research where, for example, the phrase "sexually active" can have many meanings. Precision is key, and often this means conducting unstructured formative research before constructing a questionnaire so that you can be sure of the meanings that respondents will attribute to the words used in the questions—and to be sure that your answer options, and your questions themselves, are not perceived as ridiculous.

QUESTIONS AND ANSWERS

In the 1990s, when the cultural competence movement was just gaining ground, Tervalon and Murray-Garcia (1998) argued that developing in health care workers a culturally humble attitude would be crucial to the success of the cultural competence movement. In promoting this attitude, which they termed "cultural humility," they called for "a lifelong commitment to self-evaluation and self-critique, to redressing the power imbalances in the patient-physician dynamic, and to developing mutually beneficial and nonpaternalistic clinical and advocacy partnerships with communities on behalf of individuals and defined populations" (117). This is, indeed, an ideal goal.

Cultural humility can be practiced on the large scale recommended but it also can be practiced on a smaller, local scale in the form of a general multiculturalist attitude. "The multicultural person," notes Hoopes, "is the person who has learned how to learn culture—rapidly and effectively" (1981, 10–38); or, in the words of Majumdar, it is the individual who has "mastered the knowledge and skills necessary to feel comfortable and communicate effectively with people of similar and dissimilar backgrounds, in any situation involving a group of people of diverse ethnocultural backgrounds" (1995, 2).

In becoming more multiculturally nimble, clinicians can benefit by studying the work of others, by asking considered questions in the clinic, by taking the time to learn how to ask these questions so that they make sense to the patient, by actually listening to the answers, and by otherwise familiarizing themselves with the cultural and social milieu in which patients live. Such awareness, coupled with the proper skills for cultural assessment, can allow for identifying the variables appropriate to specific cases and patient populations, and provide a more personal and empathetic understanding not only of one's patients, but of oneself.

As forecast in the concept of cultural humility, which views cultural sensitivity as much more than simple competence in a circumscribed set of cultural practices, it is not our intention here to provide a catalog of ethnic practices or a cross-cultural file in which health care workers can look up the patterned health practices of particular peoples. That approach not only leads to stereotyping, but decontextualizes human interaction and goes against the holism entailed in the culture concept. Rather the examples are meant to alert the reader to areas in which differences might be located and to the cultural processes or cultural logics that can underlie actions. This kind of alertness helps the practitioner assess individual patients with respect to various culturally based behaviors and motivations. Further, awareness that culture entails process opens the door to clinical cooperation or mutual agreement building and better patient outcomes.

Importantly, a given group's habitual actions and patterns of thought should not be noticed only when tied to pathology. As Locke notes:

> Multicultural efforts must focus on normal behaviors and wellness, rather than on abnormal behaviors and illness. Far too many efforts at meeting the needs of ethnically diverse individuals fail because they begin from a viewpoint of abnormality rather than normality. Factors such as "low self-esteem" and "self-hatred" are frequently assumed to be characteristic of ethnically diverse group members without any investigation of the basis on which such claims are made. We must also use care in how we translate research results and generalize them to populations larger than those used in the research investigations.
>
> (Locke 1992, 160)

Further, beliefs and practices related to ethnicity, although a major focus of multiculturalism, are not the only variables important to health. Harrell (1992) stresses the interconnections of ethnicity, socioeconomic status, age, and gender. It is, after all, an individual who is being treated.

FOR DISCUSSION

1. If you were caring for a patient whose language you did not speak, what would you do? What qualities would you look for in an interpreter to ensure full and forthright communication? Conversely, if you were a patient who did not understand the provider's language, what would you do? What qualities would you look for in an interpreter to ensure the type of communication desired?

2. What are some nonverbal behaviors to which health care workers should be sensitive? How might their meanings, significances, and subtleties vary cross-culturally?

3. If you took a job in a clinic far from your home that served a cultural group with which you were unfamiliar, how might you go about collecting information that would enhance your practice, enabling you to offer culturally sensitive care to patients?

4. What are the benefits of unstructured, as opposed to structured, data collection? What are the various techniques of unstructured data collection?

5. What kinds of educational activities, both for providers and for patients, might be used to encourage sensitivity and better communication in clinical settings?

CHAPTER 8

Putting Ideas into Practice: Complex Contemporary Challenges

GOAL: Draw constructively on the various concepts discussed in previous chapters in an integrative fashion to understand various health threats like HIV/AIDS, and to be able to generate ideas for future action both locally and globally.

GOAL: Understand, based on concrete examples, how health program policy makers and practitioners can productively bring cultural and social factors to bear on health issues, and how socioculturally sensitive medicine can be actualized.

Change is inevitable, and it is the hope of men and women of good will that change will be for the better—better for society and for each individual. Voluntary reform is a saner and healthier form of change than explosive measures taken as a result of abuse. It is time for analysis and reform in our medical schools and in the medical centers where interns and residents are trained if medicine—as both a science and an art—is to meet the needs of our time. Even the most thoughtful and probing analysis will be imperfect. Even the most earnestly pursued remedies will not be wholly successful. But if we cannot reach the ideal, we can move toward it. At the very least we will have had the sense and courage to try.

(Cook 1972, 211)

These words were written about 40 years ago. It is arguable whether we have moved closer to the ideal, or whether we, as a nation, even know what that ideal is. What is apparent is that our problems and our future solutions are inextricably linked to our social and cultural context, with all its difficulties, richness, and diversity.

For all of us, our social structures will determine, to a large extent, our life chances, risks, barriers, and opportunities. We all hope to be healthy, or physically and mentally able to pursue whatever we feel is worth pursuing, and we hope to be supported in our pursuits by others who care about us.

We have much in common as human beings who enter and leave this world in essentially the same way. We all die, whatever that death may mean to us and to those we love; we also develop various options for response when we become ill. Although we all face many difficulties in dealing with problems of illness, disability, and death, the diversity of our cultures and our approaches to problems testifies to human resilience and imagination.

This chapter first ties together previously presented concepts by focusing mostly on a specific health problem: AIDS, or acquired immunodeficiency syndrome. Through the prism of AIDS, we demonstrate how vital health-related needs are not addressed by the biomedical model. We illustrate the value of a culturally oriented approach—but not a culturally dominated one—for deepening our understanding in regard to widespread health challenges, of which AIDS is but one example. To set culture as determinative would impoverish our ability to institute change. The AIDS example demonstrates, however, that including culture in our purview as part of the complex human biosocial enterprises of patients and providers (and program managers, policy makers, etc.) has the opposite effect; the synergism its inclusion provides greatly enriches our capacity both to understand health problems and to act as change agents. After establishing this fact, the chapter examines the possibility of integrating biomedical with nonbiomedical approaches across the board so that our health system can more adequately meet today's challenges as well as new challenges in the future. It demonstrates that biomedicine works best when practiced in a culturally—and socially, economically, and politically—contextualized manner.

AIDS: AN OVERVIEW

First noticed by health authorities in 1981, AIDS is an end result of infection with human immunodeficiency virus or HIV. HIV is transmitted during direct physical contact, frequently through transmittal of bodily fluids such as blood or semen. It often is contracted through penetrative sexual intercourse but also may be passed on to infants in breast milk or during birth. HIV invades and destroys certain white blood cells that are essential to the proper functioning of the immune system. As the immune system breaks down, one becomes exceptionally susceptible to infectious and other diseases (like certain cancers). AIDS is the label applied to those whose immune systems have been severely challenged by HIV.

Many opportunistic infections that trouble HIV-infected individuals are caused by common viruses, fungi, bacteria, and protozoa that normally are easily disposed of by the immune system. But HIV infection disarms the immune system so that these microbes can proliferate freely, leading to frequent and severe episodes of illness. It also leads to public fear and stigma. As an HIV-positive woman commenting on the ironic nature of rejection and fearfulness of HIV-positive people on the part of the general public said: "Some people just totally freak, and [say] 'Oh my god she's HIV positive!' and 'She has AIDS!' And they're coughing all over me and gossiping at the same time. And I'm thinking, 'Don't you know that cold can kill me?' " (Sobo 1995). This chapter describes the **pandemic** (worldwide epidemic) that has caused so much death and suffering, and it shows how culture influences both risks for and responses to AIDS.

The word "**epidemic**" refers to the rapid spread of a high-prevalence disease through a given locality. But as AIDS has covered the globe so thoroughly, pandemic is a more applicable term. Some even argue that AIDS is part of a syndemic (see Chapter 2). Using the term "**syndemic**" highlights the synergy (mutually self-reinforcing action) that can exist between "two or more epidemic diseases or other disorders and the socioenvironmental context that promotes their interaction" (Singer 2009, 29).

How is AIDS part of a syndemic? Commonly, where we find high rates of AIDS we find also tuberculosis, malnutrition, and other diseases, such as herpes simplex. We also may find accompanying substance use, violence-linked injuries, and the like. Malnutrition occurs in tandem with food insufficiency and poverty, itself fueled by the loss of community members to AIDS who otherwise would be economic contributors. The syndemic concept thus draws our attention not only to disease-disease synergy but also to underlying social and environmental conditions that support—and sometimes are supported by—the synergistic coexistence of two or more epidemics at once.

Whether part of a syndemic, or a pandemic, AIDS certainly is not a plague:

> Plague is a theological idea; it refers to an event that is imputed to God. In our emotional memory, plagues are terrifying, devastating, inescapable expressions of God's wrath and judgment. Those who die in them are targets. Epidemics, no matter how serious, pale into insignificance before direct manifestations of divine anger. The word "epidemic" is a term associated with the science of public health. Epidemics are understandable aspects of nature and manageable with modern skills. People who die in them are unfortunate victims, not sinners. Epidemics come from a nonjudgmental "Nature". Plagues come from God.
>
> (Walker 1991, 3)

Recall our discussion of magic in Chapter 4. As Walker writes, "Words can heal; words can kill. In the AIDS epidemic, 'plague' is a lethal, killer word. The mindset expressed by the word underwrote the slowness and weakness of governmental action at the national, state, and local levels" when the disease was first identified (1991, 4).

AIDS TODAY

Today's most recent data (CDC 2009a) indicate that over 1.1 million people in the United States are living with HIV infections, and that one in five of these individuals do not know they have been infected. The estimated number of persons living with AIDS—the sickness acquired when HIV has broken down the immune system—was half a million; the number of people who already have died from AIDS in the United States was estimated to have been about the same.

The risk of HIV infection cuts across ethnic, class, sexual identity, and other so-called boundaries. Still, members of certain groups contract the virus more frequently than others. It is tempting to single out particular groups as **risk groups**—as bounded groups that, by virtue of some essential traits particular to the members of each, are at a high risk for AIDS. But one's risk for infection has more to do with geography and history than with ethnic, national, sexual, or other aspects of one's identity. So while aspects of identity may serve as risk markers they are not in themselves risk factors. In the following sections, we identify some of the behavioral, socioeconomic, and historical risk factors that make certain groups more vulnerable to HIV and AIDS. But first, let us look at the numbers.

The most recent data from the United States show that nearly half (47 percent) of all people living with HIV are black, one-third (34 percent) are white, and just under one in five (17 percent) are Hispanic. In terms of sex, males account for three-quarters (74 percent) of the HIV-infected population in the United States (CDC 2009a).

When compared to the world as a whole, U.S. numbers represent a drop in the bucket. Worldwide, an estimated 33 million people were living with HIV in 2007 (Joint United Nations Programme on AIDS 2008, 5). Further, the AIDS sex ratio is skewed in the United States. This is because, in the United States (as in Europe), HIV found its first stronghold in the homosexual male population. But worldwide, most HIV infections are spread through heterosexual intercourse.

And although patterns in the United States may never exactly follow suit, infections in American women are on the rise. While women accounted for an estimated 14 percent of people living with AIDS in 1992, by the end of 2005 the proportion was 23 percent (CDC 2009a). Some of the reasons for this are biological. Women involved in heterosexual intercourse (whether vaginal or anal) are generally on the receptive or receiving end, which entails a biologically higher risk for infection than penetrative partners' experience does. Rape or use of force during intercourse can exacerbate this risk. Oral contraceptive use, the use of intrauterine contraceptive devices, and vaginal or other reproductive tract infections also increase women's susceptibility to HIV (Bezemer 1992). However, ultimately, factors related to the social, political, economic, and of course cultural context of women's lives are what give shape to these **proximate** or immediate biological factors.

For instance, anal sex may be practiced by young women intent on preserving, for sociocultural reasons, their vaginal virginity. Recent data show, for instance, that 30 percent of U.S. women have engaged in this practice. The rate is highest among white non-Hispanic women (34.4 percent), and lowest among black non-Hispanic women (21.9 percent) (Leichliter et al. 2007, 1854). Hispanic women are more likely to be Catholic, a religion that favors virginity.

Further, bisexuality in men has become a major factor in transmitting HIV to women, as women may have heterosexual intercourse with bisexual men. Bisexuality in men may be more common where homosexuality is not condoned, as men will then supplement overt heterosexual relations with covert homosexual ones (see also Chapter 2).

It is generally not the one-night stand who transfers HIV to women: most are infected by steady male partners. The quality of gender relations and the structure of gender-linked power differentials increase women's risk for such infections. According to one study, men are significantly more likely than women to have lied in the negotiation of safer sex (35 percent versus 10 percent; Cochran 1989). More overt forms of submission are often seen when women lack financial resources and the things that they can buy—such as food. For instance, a study recently undertaken in Botswana and Swaziland showed that women who lack sufficient food are 70 percent less likely to feel that they have personal control in sexual relationships, 80 percent more likely to engage in survival sex, and 70 percent more likely to have unprotected sex than women with an adequate diet (Joint United Nations Programme on AIDS 2008, 11).

The good news is that the annual number of new infections overall has been on the decline. Also, in the time that has passed since the first edition of this book, deaths have slowed. This is due not only to the fact that fewer people are being infected now than during the epidemic's peak transmission years, but also to the development of AIDS drugs to combat HIV infection. Thus, although HIV/AIDS is still a leading cause of death for adults aged 25–44 in the United States, by 2006 it had dropped to sixth, down from first in the mid-1990s (Henry J. Kaiser Family Foundation 2009). It has gone, conceptually at least, from being a "death sentence" to a manageable (although still ultimately terminal) chronic disease—although access to treatment, like infection, is unevenly distributed throughout populations.

Capitalism, Modernization, and the Spread of AIDS

In Kenya, in 1989, Job Bwayo opened a free clinic for truckers near Nairobi. Blood tests revealed that 27 percent of them were HIV-positive (Conover 1993, 57). That is, more than one in four had HIV antibodies in their blood, indicating that HIV was also present. Dr. Bwayo was not surprised and may have even been relieved that things were not worse.

AIDS is **endemic** (prevalent, a common problem) in this section of Africa. Indeed, when taken together, the nations that comprise sub-Saharan Africa account for about two-thirds of all people living with HIV; 72 percent of AIDS deaths in 2007 occurred there (Joint United Nations Programme on AIDS 2008, 5). In addition to other effects, masses of orphans have been created. Kin networks that would ordinarily care for the orphans and the sick children may be structurally too weak to do so because so many family members have died off. Once-productive villages are no longer self-sufficient; labor shortages can lead to famine, increasing vulnerability to HIV infection.

AIDS's effects are staggering, especially when we consider HIV's fragility. HIV easily dies once out of the body, and it cannot go anywhere without a human host to transport it. Our bodies are the virus's chauffeurs.

Having said that, around the world HIV spreads through "a relatively restricted set of mechanisms" (Farmer 2001, 147). Modes of infection are similar everywhere. What differs from place to place, however, is the degree to which individuals are impoverished and disempowered. In some places, fatally oppressive social structural changes spurred by global capitalist interests fuel HIV's spread. For instance, in Africa, the increase in urbanization driven by the move to "modernize" after colonial agricultural schemes broke down, and the related increase in automobile, bus, and train travel as well as the growth of transcontinental trade and trucking all enabled its spread. For example, migration to cities of those seeking work and the growth of the capitalistic cash economy—which has historically denied women fair wages—led to a rise in urban prostitution (formal and informal), as urban men sought sex from women who found themselves in need of money and with no other options. High rates of untreated sexually transmitted diseases or infections (STIs) among impoverished people, and the open genital ulcers that untreated STIs usually entail, increase the likelihood for infection by giving HIV instant access to the body. When infected urban migrants return to their villages for visits, they carry HIV back into the countryside. The rapid increase of intercontinental jet travel and the movement of medical and religious missions, government representatives, business people, and especially soldiers, truckers, and tourists from one part of the globe to another gave the virus an even broader range of motion.

The spread of AIDS also seems to be fostered through increased civil strife and warfare over territory and resources that leads to blood baths and violent rape, which may increase exposure to HIV. Spread of technology has also increased use—and reuse—of injection syringes and needles and other medical equipment that is in short supply in poor nations. In addition, poor nations cannot test the safety of blood supplies for transfusions, which may also transmit HIV. Clearly, effectively combating AIDS means combating a whole range of problems raised by xmodernization processes and by the unequal distribution of wealth and health within and between nations that modernization has entailed. It means "investigating the precise mechanisms by which such forces as racism, gender inequality, poverty, war, migration, colonial heritage, coups d'état, and even structural-adjustment programs become embodied as increased risk" (Farmer 2001, 148).

AIDS PREVENTION

ABC: Practice Abstinence, Be Faithful, and Use Condoms

Individual agency may be most constrained among those most vulnerable to HIV infection, due to the pervasiveness of a cultural belief (and wish?) among program planners and funders that we each have the power to control our own health. Yet, most prevention efforts have focused on instigating individual behavior change, placing the onus for infection on the individual.

In many countries—particularly those in Africa where HIV infection rates run so high—HIV/AIDS prevention efforts center on education aimed to promote abstinence or, barring that, monogamous fidelity and condom use. The trio of strategies has been packaged as the ABC approach. In part due to the obvious problems inherent in individualizing risk when social-structural factors are key contributors, results have been mixed.

Being faithful may work for certain populations under certain economic conditions, but, as Farmer has argued, for Haiti, "unremitting hardship has clearly undermined stable patterns of union . . . by creating economic pressures to which women with dependents are particularly vulnerable" (2001, 140–41). Overall, then, condom use appears to be the most widely accepted part of this set of behavior-change advice.

Still, even when freely available, condoms often are not used. In Africa as elsewhere, this is partly because of immediate cost-benefit calculations. For example, "truck stop girls," who often are destitute, know that men will pay more for sex without condoms (Maternowska 2009).

Local knowledge about condoms also comes into play. Importantly, local knowledge is shaped by a long-term legacy of colonial and capitalist oppression and exploitation. African truckers interviewed by Ted Conover introduced him to an innkeeper named Bora at one of their stops, and among the news she had for them as they relaxed in the pub was a story about a man who had recently died of AIDS: "It turned out that when the authorities went to the house, they found dozens of packages of unused condoms [with] dates that had expired! Knowing murmurs circled the table, and I asked Francis [a trucker] to explain. 'These condoms, when they are too old, contain germs,' he said. 'And that's how he got AIDS'" (1993, 68).

AIDS-related myths are in no way constrained to Africa, but they do seem more common among the disenfranchised. People of color in the United States and elsewhere have reported that AIDS was invented by the Army as part of a germ-warfare scheme. To dismiss such notions out of hand could validate people's beliefs that the health care system does not care about them and cannot be trusted (DeParle 1990; Herek and Capitanio 1994). Commonsense beliefs must be fought with commonsense logic.

Poor-quality condoms also are not unique to Africa. And their quality probably did not start out as poor. But hot weather and shipping delays can lead to latex deterioration. Problems also can result because clinicians fail or do not have time to provide clients with full instructions on how condoms are to be cared for, used, and taken off.

Another problem that educators might address concerns people's propensity to focus on condoms' contraceptive function over and above their value for blocking HIV transmission and the transmission of other pathogens. Therefore, using condoms when trying to build a family may be seen as making little sense, especially when one's culture places a high value on children. Alternately, using condoms when one or both sex partners has undergone sterilization or uses another family-planning method can seem redundant when condoms are linked in the mind so strongly with contraception. Moreover, consistent condom use can be hard to maintain within regular partnerships, especially when these partnerships are multiple and concurrent, as they often are in high-prevalence populations (Potts et al. 2008).

On the other hand, sex-positive information on how condoms can enhance sex (e.g., by making erections last longer) and instruction on how to incorporate condoms into the sex act have been shown to offset negative attitudes toward condoms (e.g., Tanner and Pollack 1988). Further, broad-based health ideals can be brought into play in AIDS interventions, as can the idea of staying healthy for the good of one's family. For example, a recent effort to reach North San Diego's Latino population with HIV risk-reduction information and services centered on comprehensive male health concerns in general, including hypertension and diabetes screenings, rather than focusing only on

HIV/AIDS in particular. Resulting increases in condom use and HIV testing were found (Martínez-Donate et al. 2009).

While improved interventions help increase condom use, full buy-in is unlikely, for reasons reviewed earlier. Further, impoverished people and members of disenfranchised minority groups also need better access to health care services, which will lead to better overall health. Better health will make it harder for HIV to gain a foothold in the body, and improved health care delivery will lead individuals to be more trusting of the system's AIDS prevention recommendations.

As the example of AIDS shows us, in order to fully grasp the multifaceted nature of a health threat, and to promote education, positive attitudes, healthy behaviors, and effective care, it is essential to consider, understand, and leverage the connections between social and cultural factors and illness and care. This requires an integrated approach to the human experience of health and illness as well as an expansion of the biomedical model to include social, cultural, political, and economic factors.

GENDER AND HIV PREVENTION: A U.S. CASE STUDY

As the foregoing suggests, HIV prevention strategies are implemented in cultural context and gender expectations are part of every culture. Yet the impact that cultural constructions of gender have on HIV acquisition rates varies. This has to do not only with variations in gender itself, but also—and perhaps moreover—with variation among other sociocultural factors. So, for example, rather than all women being affected equally by HIV, black and Hispanic women account for 82 percent of all women living with HIV/AIDS in the United States (CDC 2008a). In this section, we concentrate on the situation for disadvantaged urban black women in the United States— the group with which we have the most experience.

HIV infection rates are higher than average among urban black women—this despite the fact that, overall, black women seem to take fewer sexual risks than white women (e.g., Leichliter et al. 2007, 1854; Lewis and Watters 1989; Weinberg and Williams 1988; see also Wilson 1987; Worth 1990).

If taking fewer overt risks, why then are black women disproportionately represented? As in impoverished nations, the conditions of life in the U.S. inner-city make condomless penetrative sex more likely to lead to HIV infection among those who live there than, say, among those who are part of less disadvantaged social networks. Economic oppression (and the effects of this on gender relations), substandard health care, the frequency of injecting drug use, high rates of untreated STIs, and other typical inner-city and poverty-related conditions—all linked to higher order political-economic arrangements that benefit the rich—exacerbate the effects that unsafe sex practices have on the rate of HIV transmission among poor urban black men and women.

There are also cultural reasons for the disparities in HIV transmission rates among black people, shaped as they are by social-structural arrangements. Some cultural factors supporting HIV transmission given these arrangements have to do with sexual and reproductive expectations. As among most peoples, cultural norms for sexuality here differ between men and women. Men are expected to have active extraconjugal sex lives while women are not. This is generally traced to man's lack of economic opportunity and his related dependence on favorable peer evaluations (Anderson 1990; Liebow 1967). William Oliver (1989) explains the "complex of values and norms that characterize the way many lower-class Black males define manhood"—a complex that includes "the tough guy and the player-of-women images"—as a "cultural adaptation to white racism" and a "compensatory adaptation" (260, 261). Following Hannerz, who wrote in the 1960s, Oliver calls this complex "compulsive masculinity" (Hannerz 1969, as cited on 261). Not much has changed.

Men are often eager to sire offspring as proof of their heterosexual activity, and women can have children to please and bind men—to establish kinship-type links with them and their kin. Childbearing also can be a way of trying to improve one's status: Each child born holds the promise of achieving great things and of reflecting well on the mother as well as of being a source of joy and of unconditional love.

Knowing that the supply of marriageable or employed men is very small, some women choose to build families and network connections without the perceived burden of a husband/boyfriend. But unprotected sex, necessary in many cases for male support (whether social, emotional, or financial) and always needed for conception, entails HIV and STI risks.

OPTIMISM AND RISK MIS/PERCEPTION

As Fischoff and colleagues have argued, the "choice of an option depends upon all of its features, not just its risk" (1981, 134). The risk of HIV infection and so of AIDS is just one of many risks faced daily by impoverished urban minority women. Under such conditions, the benefits of heterosexual interaction and of possible pregnancy and childbearing outweigh the risk of disease when not risking this could lead to more immediate consequences such as verbal or physical abuse, the loss of a partner, or childlessness. All of these consequences involve concrete hardship as well as lowered status and damaged self-esteem.

Relevant cultural knowledge and information about culture-specific role expectations is essential for developing predictions of when and how specific kinds of AIDS risk denial will occur, and strategies to combat this denial and so to reduce risk behaviors and control the spread of AIDS. No matter what one's objective risk level is, in the context of mainstream U.S. culture, believing or indicating that one is at risk for AIDS would involve admitting one's failure to live up to standards for prudent sexual (or drug-related) behavior (the shortcomings of these standards notwithstanding). Because such an admission could have dire effects on self-esteem, identity, and status, many people maintain what Weinstein (1989) has called **optimistically biased** AIDS risk denial. That is, they play down or ignore their own risks for HIV infection; they fail to apply to themselves or to **personalize** messages regarding AIDS risks.

Frightening thoughts of one's susceptibility, social marginality, and impending physical and, moreover, social death need not be confronted if one's AIDS risk is denied. Further, denying this allows a person to preserve her own self-esteem and status just as admitting it by using condoms can lower self-esteem. This is because denying one's risk for AIDS involves denying that one engages in stigmatized practices, including unwise partnering choices.

By denying risk, people not only can preserve but also can raise their status and self-esteem, as denying one's own risk implicitly—and sometimes explicitly—involves asserting that others are at a higher risk for the problem than oneself. Indeed, people often report that their peers' risk levels for negative outcomes like AIDS are higher than their own. In part, this is because people tend to compare themselves to stereotypic images of those who take few or no self-protective actions; that is, we compare ourselves to high-risk individuals rather than to our actual peers (Weinstein 1982, 1989). So, for instance, a person may say (as a real research participant once did): "I know four brothers (all drug abusers) who have AIDS but I don't do what they do and besides they live in a different neighborhood" (Kinsey 1994;

83; parentheses in original). Similarly, people may use negative HIV test results to support their self-affirming contentions that they were not at risk for contracting the virus. The cognitive or thought process of optimistic bias seems to have no link with a person's actual risk level (Hansen, Hahn, and Wolkenstein 1990; Weinstein 1989).

Rather, optimistic bias has a strong tie to the degree to which a condition is stigmatized (Prohaska, Albrecht, and Levy 1990). It also has a strong tie to a risk's perceived preventability (Weinstein 1989). As Weinstein writes, "The more preventable the hazard, the greater the threat to self-esteem" (1989, 157), and the greater the threat to self esteem, the more useful optimistic bias can be. This makes the job of the AIDS prevention counselor in the United States even more difficult, as AIDS is seen as preventable by many Americans.

COMPLEMENTING CONDOMS: MALE CIRCUMCISION AND STI TREATMENT

It is in part for reasons such as those explained previously that Potts and colleagues (2008) argue condoms are most helpful in stemming infections spread mainly through sex work, which is the case in, for instance, Thailand. Potts's group also finds them useful for certain high-risk groups such as men who have sex with men. But their review of the literature suggests that condoms are not the answer for nations (and populations) where the epidemic is **generalized** rather than limited to narrow subpopulations. The low effectiveness of condoms for stemming the spread of HIV under generalized epidemic conditions has to do with the fact that, despite all efforts, condom use levels remain too low overall. What, then, can be of help?

Randomized controlled trials in Africa have shown that HIV acquisition by men can be reduced by about 60 percent with male circumcision (Bailey and Mehta 2009). Epidemiological models predict that over the next 20 years male circumcision might prevent up to 5.7 million new infections and 3 million deaths (Potts et al. 2008, 750). Ecological studies have shown that HIV infections are less common in regions where circumcision is practiced (Ngalande et al. 2006). When fewer men who have sex with women are infected, eventually, so too will fewer women acquire HIV.

What is going on here to support direct protection of men? Simply put, "the circumcised penis is covered by a thick layer of keratin, whereas the inner mucosal surface of the foreskin has no such protective layer" (Ngalande et al. 2006, 377). Further, the lining of the inner foreskin has a high density of the kinds of cells that HIV targets. These features are what put uncircumcised men—men with intact foreskins—at risk for infection (377–78)—particularly where people are not afforded clean running water to wash with, as in many economically poor regions. Notably, these uncircumcised men can be at risk for other sexually transmitted infections, too; and having an STI such as genital herpes increases one's risk for acquiring HIV. For this reason, treatment of other STIs is seen as key to effective HIV prevention by public health experts (Potts et al. 2008).

The biological reality of HIV vulnerability is one thing. The cultural acceptability of such prevention plans as STI treatment or male circumcision is another. To take the latter, for example: Male circumcision is a key feature of Jewish and Muslim identity. Circumcision also is practiced routinely on newborn boys by pediatricians in the United States. But in other populations, the practice is viewed by some as unnecessary and by others as barbaric, damaging, dangerous, and stigmatizing.

In light of this, a male circumcision acceptability study was undertaken in Malawi in the early 2000s, when only 20 percent of males had been circumcised. It, led to the promising finding that many would welcome male circumcision if its provision was safe, affordable, and confidential. Because in Malawi penis hygiene is a cultural concern—cleaning the penis is considered an essential task during bathing and after sex—a focus on the hygienic benefits of the practice would be relevant. So would information pertaining to the sexual benefits of circumcision. Further, as most Malawi ethnic groups are matrilineal, involving women in male circumcision campaigns there would be prudent. However elsewhere, for instance in Botswana, men may be key decision makers (Ngalande et al. 2006).

HIV TESTING

One context for education regarding strategies such as condom use or even circumcision is during voluntary HIV counseling and testing. The time when a test is administered or results shared with a patient can be a "teachable moment" when risks are assessed and education offered. This also is true when results are positive; although when that is the case education often must be delayed in order to be effective, due to the shock that a positive result can entail. Indeed, voluntary counseling and testing has become a well-established part of HIV transmission prevention as well as being a pathway to care worldwide (Potts et al. 2008).

In the United States, where heretofore one-fourth of all people infected with HIV seem not to have known it, the CDC recently made a landmark shift in policy, calling for routine HIV testing among adults, adolescents, and pregnant women. Testing still is voluntary, but rather than having to self-consciously opt in, thereby drawing attention to one's risk-related behaviors (or those of one's partner/s), people now have the option instead to decline the test offer (Bayer and Fairchild 2006). "Routinization" (Sobo et al. 2008) both partly de-stigmatizes HIV/AIDS and streamlines the whole testing process by treating it like any other form of medical screening. This makes it easier not only for patients (who also can access care earlier if infection is detected) but also for providers. And health care organizations and payers benefit, too: Routine testing is cost effective (Sanders et al. 2005).

Still, and although attitudes slowly are changing, voluntary counseling and testing is not without challenges. Many people never entertain the thought of being screened for HIV infection. Many simply do not see themselves as being "at risk," often for reasons such as those discussed earlier. For others, when resources are scarce and treatment options therefore limited, testing may not seem to offer useful information.

For those who do acknowledge their risk for having been infected, the social risks of testing can be too high: Sometimes, even being seen going for an HIV test may be stigmatizing. HIV is commonly transmitted through sexual contact. It is sometimes considered as a punishment for culturally unacceptable forms of sexual expression—or as implying that one's social relationships are in a poor state. HIV/AIDS therefore often carries a culturally constructed **stigma** or mark of disgrace (see Goffman 1959). People may need to avoid stigmatization to protect their families—and themselves—from dishonor or even violent attacks.

Clinicians, for their part, may make assumptions about a person's risk status and never even offer the HIV test, even when risk factors such as sexually transmitted diseases, substance use, or blood transfusions are in patients' medical records. Alternately, they may avoid it (when they can rationalize doing so) due to the paperwork and follow-up burden that it can entail (Sobo et al. 2008).

The ramifications of a positive diagnosis with HIV or AIDS can be enormous. Those who get tested—and return for their results—often find the **lexicon** or vocabulary that clinicians use confusing, and this can lead to mistaken interpretations of results. For instance, tested individuals sometimes understand positive results as "good" or as indicating that one is free of HIV, when the opposite is the case. Further, people who think that they have "passed" the HIV test sometimes equate their perceived negative status with immunity, and this can lead to an attitude of carelessness or even to an increase in risk behavior (Kurth and Hutchinson 1989). Those involved in testing and counseling should concentrate on clearly conveying meanings by translating medical jargon into plain English (or other appropriate languages), and they should double-check clients' understandings to make sure that they are correct.

POSITIVE RESULTS

If test results are positive, the testee must adjust to his or her new status. The individual's psychological reaction is influenced by his or her own cultural beliefs and the perceived cultural beliefs of members of his or her social networks.

Individual identity constructions affect how people deal with HIV seropositivity. As Borden has noted, "HIV seropositivity is likely to threaten existing interpretations of self, others, life experience, and anticipated future" (1991, 438); in other words, a positive HIV test may entail a need to revise one's life history, and this can be devastating. In some cases, one must adjust to fears about infecting partners and children, or in abandoning them through death. Coping with HIV or AIDS also involves grieving for and ultimately accepting the potential loss of one's future as well as accepting the uncertainty that comes with the disease. Those who learn they are HIV-positive must then also deal with the hope of treatment.

TO TELL OR NOT TO TELL?

In light of the foregoing, it will be clear that the seropositive weigh a number of factors to determine whether or not and to whom they will disclose their status. These factors are intimately linked with cultural assumptions about HIV and AIDS.

Some of the main reasons for nondisclosure include not wanting to worry or upset others, fear of discrimination, fear of disrupting relationships, emotional self-protection, feeling that the person told would have little beneficial to offer, a lack of closeness with the individual, and the desire to conceal one's homosexuality (Hays et al. 1993). Although these findings were gathered prior to the widespread use of antiretroviral therapy for HIV/AIDS, all indications are that nondisclosure reasoning remains much the same. Further, the basic cultural logic of non/disclosure is relevant to other chronic conditions as well.

AIDS TREATMENTS

BIOMEDICAL CARE FOR HIV/AIDS

Before the middle 1990s, a diagnosis of HIV infection or AIDS was not a diagnosis that one could do much about. Effective treatments were not yet on the market. However, scientists had discovered that certain pharmaceuticals were effective in limiting or inhibiting HIV's ability to reproduce. In short, these were antiretrovirals (HIV is a retrovirus—one with RNA rather than DNA at its core). Soon, scientific findings confirmed that antiretroviral therapy (ART) was highly effective or "highly active" (HA) against HIV/AIDS when three or four antiretroviral drugs were used in combination: Highly active antiretroviral therapy (HAART) was born. HAART cannot cure HIV/AIDS but what it can do, quite well when taken as directed, is slow the virus's pace of replication. The combination or "cocktail" of various forms of ART helps to ensure against the development of strains of HIV that are resistant to a single antiretroviral. Side effects can be severe and medication regimens confusing. Costs can be prohibitive. Notwithstanding, effective treatment does now exist and many people living with HIV/AIDS in fact have viral loads so low as to be undetectable through common testing methods.

Others, however, have been denied access to treatment. Some in health care held the opinion that treatment in conditions of poverty would not work because patients living under such conditions could not adhere to a recommended care plan. Nothing has been further from the truth, when patients have been well supported—including with a regular, secure drug supply. HAART adherence rates in countries such as Malawi have been just as good as in financially rich countries such as the United States, if not better (Harries, Schouten, and Libamba 2006). Indeed, as members of Partners in Health have shown in projects in Haiti and elsewhere—for tuberculosis (including the resistant kind) as well as for HIV/AIDS—with additional nutritional support and a little bit of financial aid for destitute patients, much can be accomplished (e.g., Farmer 2001).

This is not to say that adherence to a medication regimen is easy, even when supported. In addition to side effects, and the reality that in some populations the fact that one is taking HIV/AIDS medications must be hidden due to stigmatization, there also can be challenges related to inequity in access to care. That is, when one member of a close social network is considered eligible for treatment—for instance a pregnant mother—but another—for instance her partner—is not, due simply to treatment program narrowness, pill sharing can occur. As a result of **pill sharing** (in which everyone might get some pills, but at lower-than-would-be-prescribed doses), HIV can actually spread further and evolve drug-resistant strains. In addition, providers may make poor decisions on a patient's behalf, lacking the full story about where his or her pills are going.

HIV seropositivity is not generally one's worst problem if one is poor: There are often other sick people in the family as well as children to feed and rent to be paid. Gender expectations complicate things further. Because of gender expectations, like most mainstream women, poor urban women with HIV or AIDS often feel that they must take care of others before they take care of themselves.

In the United States, women frequently find it easier to bring a sick child to the doctor than to go in for their own appointments (and while some clinics have recently tried to group appointments for patient convenience, adults and children often must go to different clinics, on different days). Clinicians are often more sympathetic toward pediatric AIDS cases than they are toward sick women: one researcher found that while "many service providers, professionals, and volunteers attend the funeral of a baby dead from AIDS, not one of them is present at the mother's funeral" (Ward 1993b, 60).

Mothers or not, quality health care often is beyond reach for poor people infected with HIV. In addition to health care that often is not covered by what little insurance (if any) a poor person has, money often is unavailable for transportation to appointments, child care, and so forth. Drugs for HIV-related conditions can be prohibitively expensive. There are also problems when heterosexuals are sent for treatment to centers that cater instead to gay men, or vice versa.

Beside all this, people of color may suffer from racism in the health care system (see Chapter 2). It is manifested in cursory physical examinations, inadequate bed assignments, delayed admissions, and assumptions of noncompliance. Racism often overlaps with discrimination against the poor, and it influences the adoption, implementation, and administration of health policies that negatively affect the lives of lower-income people (Hutchinson 1993; Barr 2008).

NONBIOMEDICAL HEALING

When biomedical care is not available, it is our responsibility to make it so (Farmer 2005). But before this happens, what is a person with HIV/AIDS to do? And even when available, biomedicine cannot answer the question "why me." Further, practiced narrowly, it cannot heal social problems. If seeking a substitute for biomedicine when it is unavailable, or healing that will supplement or complement biomedical care, what are one's options?

The answers are many and varied, although across the board they attempt to provide people with a meaningful way to handle the existential questions and human suffering entailed in human sickness. One thing that substitute systems do provide is help in understanding why a particular person contracts HIV/AIDS when another just like him or her does not. In Haiti, for instance, in certain cases an infection with HIV may be explained as having been sent by an enemy, using supernatural means. So sometimes people consult Voodoo, or Vodoun, priests.

Vodoun is Haiti's traditional indigenous religion. A hybrid of African and Catholic traditions, Vodoun, like any religion, provides explanations for misfortune, and its rituals have healing power. Many people of Haitian as well as other Caribbean origins living in the United States practice diffused and adapted versions of this religion. In the islands, too, a large number of similarly generated religious hybrids exist and, among other things, they all have healing functions.

If AIDS has been sent as a hex or curse sometimes the priest works to return the misfortune to the person who arranged to send it. He or she also works to cure the infection. Often, this entails holding public ceremonies to please the spirit world. Such ceremonies generally consist of much drumming, dancing, singing, and praying, and food is offered to the gods. Participants often are possessed by spirits enticed to visit by the congregation's festivities. Priests also work private rituals for the sick. Sometimes, they mix medicines from herbs and other ingredients.

This example demonstrates that people will use their traditional health beliefs to explain and manage, or try to manage, modern health threats. Research concerning responses to AIDS among Mexican Americans and Mexicans living near the U.S.-Mexico border provides an other example of this (Rivera 1990). Many Mexicans and Mexican Americans subscribe to the healing system called *Curanderismo*, in which indigenous healers known as *curanderos* (male) or *curanderas* (female) are consulted. Curanderismo provides explanations and treatments for numerous health problems. Treatments include plant-based medicines, prayer, or magical rites such as the burning of candles.

While interviews revealed that some curandero/as felt that they could not treat AIDS, others had devised treatment plans modeled on traditional treatments for illnesses involving symptoms similar to those exhibited with AIDS. However, they did not see AIDS as related to these illnesses. And they did not explain AIDS as the result of witchcraft or sorcery. Instead, the healers considered AIDS as a new communicable disease brought on by excess pollution in the body, an imbalance of acids, or the body's invasion by *mal aire*, or evil (bad, tainted) air. Those who thought it incurable recommended praying to St. Lazarus, who was raised from the dead, as they would for people with any incurable illness (Rivera 1990).

People the world over pick and choose from all available systems— traditional and modern, folk and professional—when devising their therapy regimens. People living with HIV/AIDS in San Francisco might combine biomedical attention with Chinese herbalism or Christian prayer; those in Santa Fe, New Mexico, might add Curanderismo and New Age crystal therapy to their biomedical treatment regimes. In other words, integrative medicine already is being practiced at the grass roots. Therefore, as long as CAM is not used as a substitute for or instead of proven therapies, inclusion into health care regimens could provide cultural support and comfort and augment healing.

INTEGRATION OF HEALTH CARE MODALITIES

Many factors block such expansion and integration. Probably one of the strongest barriers to integration is the primacy of the scientific model, which, even with its limitations, is necessary and vital. Without it, we would have no progress or advancement through technology, and no real understanding of biological and physical processes. Due to the strong focus on the scientific aspect of medicine, however, there has been until recently very little research demonstrating the efficacy or benefits of nonbiomedical therapeutic interventions either alone or in combination with biomedical treatments, and only limited attempts at incorporation of alternative values or care into biomedical regimens.

JOINT COLLABORATION

While not many success stories have yet happened, one is by now an anthropological classic. That is the story of the Navajo-Cornell Medical School joint project (Adair, Deuschle, and Barnett 1988 [1972]). In this project, an interdisciplinary team designed and administered an experimental health program on the Navajo reservation in Arizona, in partnership with the Navajo Tribal Council and the Tribal Health Committee. From the beginning, contact between all parties was respectful and honest. The project was jointly funded (the Tribal Council had contributed 10,000 1953 dollars); ownership and all that it entails—including responsibility, accountability, and pride in a job well done—was jointly distributed.

Cultural sensitivity infused the project and fueled its appeal. The clinic was blessed by a medicine man on its opening day, and local concerns rather than what outsiders defined as problems were prioritized. Clinicians built local forms of social organization into medical record keeping practices, for example, recording clanship (119). In addition, native practitioners were consulted for ideas and opinions from the initial days of the project's inception. Of course, from the Navajo point of view, the clinic was incorporated by native medical practitioners such that traditional and biomedical systems became integrated.

To diagnose illness, Navajo shamans go into trance and practice hand trembling, in which hand movements produce and erase designs in the sand, which are then interpreted or read. After the clinic's establishment, native diagnosticians could, on the basis of the signs, refer patients to the clinic just as they could, on the basis of the signs, recommend particular traditional healing strategies, or even that the patient combine both types of response. Many clinic patients utilized both medical systems, and the project clinicians never discouraged this; some Navajo clinic workers had themselves been trained in traditional healing ways (e.g., 91).

In the words of Adair and his colleagues, this integration reflects "a recognition that illness in the individual involves many components needing treatment and both systems are necessary for complete treatment" (1988, 170). So, for example, a man with appendicitis had a healing ceremony performed after his appendectomy operation. He explained that the ceremony would help the incision to heal.

Further, it provided a ritualized means of reentering his community after the hospital stay; his relatives, neighbors, and friends attended the ceremony, wished him well, and expressed pleasure at his presence back home.

In addition to simple sensitivity to cultural differences and respect for native ways, the emphasis of the project on direct Navajo participation accounts to a large degree for the project's success.

INTEGRATION OF BIOMEDICINE IN THE COMMUNITY

As the collaborative Navajo example shows, the need to expand the role of biomedical practitioners, especially those in primary care, does not actually entail an impossible workload or extended study and responsibility. Practitioners are already politically oriented through professional interests. As they interact with families and communities, the workload entailed by cultural sensitivity may be shared, and such sharing may improve relationships and mutual understanding among patients and practitioners. The term "patient advocate" thereby becomes more meaningful and patients may also become "practitioner advocates."

The concept of health and illness, in addition, must be expanded to include culturally relevant definitions that are demonstrably related to treatment outcomes. As demonstrated in Chapter 2, many health problems are linked to poverty and social and environmental conditions such that curative medical treatment provides only a momentary palliative. For example, a child's rash might clear up with ointment. But if the rash is caused by exposure to some kind of toxin in the child's play environment and the toxin is not removed from that environment, the rash will keep reappearing. The old saying that "an ounce of prevention is worth a pound of cure" speaks to this problem. In many cases, the ounce of prevention needed has to do with improving life environments through the development of community resources, including education, provision of services, and community empowerment.

This point is clearly seen in a brief review of some of the work of Caroll Behrhorst, a Kansas physician who worked for nearly 30 years in Guatemala. Behrhorst founded a small clinic and teaching center in Chimaltenango. In addition to on-site and outreach health work, carried out by local people trained by Behrhorst, the center also instituted agricultural development programs with the aim of increasing people's living standards and self-sufficiency.

As Behrhorst tells it, his emphasis on community development grew from a realization that "I was trying to empty an ocean of disease and malfunction with a medical teaspoon" (1993, 58). After treating children suffering from malaise, puffy eyes, swollen feet, discolorations of the skin, diarrhea, and coughing, Behrhorst "realized that, no mater how many times we treated [the youngsters], they would never be healthy until basic changes were made in the village" (58).

The changes began when a Peace Corps volunteer who had gained the trust of people living in Chimaltenango and the surrounding villages began to introduce new farming methods. Later, money was lent from the clinic's operating funds for families to invest in laying chickens. Soon, people had more protein in their diets. Another group borrowed money to buy some land, and another formed a weaving and marketing cooperative. As cash began to flow, the loans were repaid. The health of the villagers improved dramatically once they had a firm economic base to sustain them. As Behrhorst wrote, "What started as curing the sick broadened into a general community program geared to activities that the residents want and need and that result in self-empowerment" (60–61).

All along, Behrhorst and the local people worked to make the clinic independent rather than to allow the Chimaltenango project to remain dependent on outside aid and foreign clinicians. Behrhorst said, "If we outsiders do not plan ways of doing ourselves out of a job we are probably not doing the job at all" (1993, 61). In 1975, the Chimaltenango project was identified by the World Health Organization (WHO) as one of 10 worldwide models for effective health promotion, and later WHO declarations and agendas were built to a large degree on the model Behrhorst and his Guatemalan colleagues had developed (Luecke 1993, xviii).

Similar programs have since been put into place in other parts of the world. The work of Partners in Health (PIH) serves as a good example. Founded in 1987, PIH exists to serve the poor in solidarity: "When a person in Peru, or Siberia, or rural Haiti falls ill, PIH uses all of the means at our disposal to make them well—from pressuring drug manufacturers, to lobbying policy makers, to providing medical care and social services. Whatever it takes. Just as we would do if a member of our own family—or we ourselves—were ill" (Partners in Health 2009).

Partners in Health is the English translation of the name of a community-based health project, *Zanmi Lasante*, started in Haiti in 1985 to serve the peasants of Cange, many of whom had been displaced from elsewhere when flooded out by a dam built for the benefit of American-owned agribusinesses and, in faraway Port au Prince, for a small group of wealthy Haitians as well as foreign-owned assembly plants (Kidder 2003, 37–38; Farmer 1992). One founder, Paul Farmer, then working toward both a PhD and MD and now a specialist in infectious disease, was greatly interested at the time in the relationship between health behavior and cultural models, such as those regarding blood, germs, and sorcery. He expected these to explain patterns of, for instance, nonadherence to a treatment plan.

Despite the great power that culture holds, to his surprise Farmer found that the Haitian peasants' adherence to biomedical treatment for tuberculosis differed not according to whether or how much people believed the disease had been sent to them with sorcery but rather according to how supported they were in their treatment regimen—whether they received home visits and small cash stipends for food, transportation to the clinic, and child care (see Kidder 2003, 34–35). Stemming from this, Farmer realized that what people do with their beliefs—how they deploy them to give voice to the dilemmas in which they have been placed by political, social, and economic history—is key. The legacy of social, economic, and political suffering Haitians expressed in stories told about being ensorcelled or how AIDS was sent to their island by the U.S. government were what needed attending to (e.g., Farmer 1999). Doing that—really listening to the underlying stories that cultural beliefs express—is one true expression of cultural sensitivity.

Of course sensitive clinical care alone would not heal the ailments expressed through patients' stories. For that, true partnerships were needed—partnerships with patients but also with the community as a whole, for instance in terms of building sustainability by providing training for local people so that they might staff the clinic, and in terms of determining priority programs. Moreover, because the community was, like all communities, whether rural or urban, part of a global system, other partnerships had to be created—partnerships with drug companies, for instance, so that treatments for HIV/AIDS and tuberculosis could be made accessible to those who most needed but could least afford them—and partnerships with those involved in "development" such as created the detrimental dam, so that peasant needs, too, would be part of future "development" equations. True devotion to the concept and actualization of "partnership" is what has made PIH's work such a success. This philosophy, and the fact that PIH's Haitian clinics were rurally located, made PIH-affiliated services indispensible in the aftermath of Haiti's devastating January 2010 earthquake; indeed, PIH took the lead with its care model, at the Haitian government's own request (Smith and Smith 2010).

Community-oriented health programs exist not only overseas but also in the United States. For example, in one classic case, people living in a predominantly poor black community on the west side of Chicago formed a voluntary community organization to address health problems (McKnight 1993).

The first problem confronted was that of a lack of access to local hospitals. After this hurdle was surmounted, the health status of community members did not improve. Hospital medical records revealed that the main health problems of the community were not, in fact, the kinds that are best solved through curative medicine. The most common reasons for the hospitalization of community members were, in order of frequency, automobile accidents, interpersonal attacks, accidents (other than those involving autos), bronchial ailments, alcoholism, drug-related problems, and dog bites. This startled community members, who had in effect succumbed to medicalization, assuming that their health problems could be solved by biomedicine alone. McKnight, who chronicled their progress, saw this as an important step in the health consciousness of this community to recognize that modern medical systems are frequently dealing with maladies that are social problems rather than diseases (1993, 221).

After considering their options, the people in the organization decided to start at the bottom of the list. Dog bites accounted for about 4 percent of all emergency room visits. Dogs—including wild ones—were indeed a neighborhood nuisance. The organization let it be known through neighborhood block associations that they would pay a bounty or reward for each captured dog. The neighborhood youth thought this a great game, and in one month's time 160 dogs were captured. Emergency room admissions for dog bites went down accordingly. Not only had the group learned that their own actions could improve health, but they also were involving community youth in positive, community-building activities.

After their initial success, the group targeted automobile accidents for reduction. They first sought to find out where most accidents occurred. They plotted three months' worth of accident data on a map of the neighborhood to locate the most dangerous areas. In one area, six people had been injured and one killed. This area was the entrance to a department store. The organization contacted the owner and successfully negotiated for a change in the entrance's layout.

Bronchial problems were the third issue addressed. The group learned that such problems were linked to nutrition and concluded that people in the neighborhood did not eat enough fresh fruit and vegetables. They could not afford to. Several group members noted that greenhouses might be built on the flat roofs of neighborhood dwellings. And, as McKnight recalls, "a number of fascinating things began to happen" (1993, 224).

The greenhouses worked: They provided cheap fruit and vegetables that people could sell to generate income as well as eat. Further, the greenhouses insulated people's dwellings and absorbed heat that might otherwise have leaked out of the rooftops.

The community organization owned a retirement home for the elderly. One day, one of the residents wandered into the greenhouse and started to work there on a regular basis. Other residents joined her. The attitude of these residents changed: "They were excited. They had found a function and a purpose. The greenhouse had become a tool to empower the elderly—it enabled discarded people to become productive" (McKnight 1993, 225).

Overall, the group's mission involved removing the underlying causes of disease or injury when they could, and adding health-promoting options into the community when possible. McKnight explains, "Converting medical problems into community issues proved central to health improvement [and] increased the organization's vitality and power" (1993, 226). The health actions instigated led away from overdependence on the local hospital and toward self-sufficient or low-consumption health strategies. In light of the ever-increasing costs of providing clinical care, and the increasing fragmentation of communities throughout the United States, the promotion of similar groups' health- and community-building activities seems a sound investment.

As a final example of such an approach, take the efforts of the Tohono O'odham Nation of Arizona, who have among the highest diabetes rates in the world. Several generations ago the Tohono O'odham lost their right to the region's water when the river that their farming lifestyle depended upon was diverted to service nonnative farmers upstream. At that time, and in fact until the 1960s, no known case of diabetes existed among the Tohono O'odham. However, when they lost their livelihood and the cultural ways that went with it, they also lost the means to good health: physical activity, a balanced diet, and a hopeful outlook. Indeed, chronic stress such as that engendered by the historical trauma this group has lived through itself can provoke the overproduction of stress hormones that have been linked to diabetes (California Newsreel 2008a).

Today, more than half of all Tohono O'odham adults have been diagnosed with type 2 (adult onset) diabetes—as have increasing numbers of Tohono O'odham children. Because diabetes rates now are so high in this group, they have become favorites for biomedical research. However, rather than simply submitting to academic desires to conduct genetic testing in support of an individualized, gene-based understanding of why they are more likely to have diabetes than other populations, or otherwise offering themselves as human test subjects for others' research projects, members of the Tohono O'odham Nation came together to form Tohono O'odham Community Action, or TOCA, a community-based organization dedicated to re-creating a sustainable, healthy culture (http://www.tocaonline.org/Home.html). TOCA promotes cultural renewal and the empowerment this entails as key to the physical health and overall wellness of the people.

At present, TOCA has four primary program areas: basket weaving, traditional foods, youth/elder outreach, and traditional arts and culture. All are intertwined. The traditional foods program area, however, is perhaps most directly related diabetes abatement. It emphasizes not only healthy eating but also seeks to reteach traditional farming skills, such as were lost when the river was diverted, through school programs and other outreach efforts. In support of this, TOCA strives to revitalize the cultural aspects of Tohono O'odham foodways, using native traditions in the context in which they were meant to be used rather than as, for instance, performing a ground-blessing ceremony on a stage. TOCA also helps to support traditional farming efforts by creating markets for the foods so grown, including via its Web site.

Rather than simply endorsing and working to ensure access to the current clinical model of diabetes care, which of course is important, TOCA emphasizes a community-based model of holistic diabetes intervention. It acknowledges the material roots of the community's culture and therefore of its overall health. In this, TOCA also understands the community as part of a larger system. Ultimately, it aims to address the structural causes of unemployment and poverty and so of ill health among the Tohono O'odham people. Advocacy of the kind that led to the Arizona Water Rights Settlement Act, which went into effect in 2008 but was over 30 years in the making (Archibold 2008), has been a crucial part of this process.

SOCIOCULTURAL MEDICINE?

The models subscribed to and promoted by PIH, TOCA, and others are laudable and workable. But they are community based. What about clinical medicine? Can culture, and all that it entails, be quite as useful there? Throughout this book, we have argued that it can—and that good clinicians do this anyhow. On that topic, here is Robert Hahn:

> If the healing process invariably requires an understanding of different perceptions of the world; if understandings of sickness are culturally given and organized; if sickness is caused in part by social organization and social relations; if healing depends on effective relationships across cultural boundaries; if, in other words, social and cultural conditions and events underlie the healing process, then healers—Biomedical and others—unwittingly make anthropological assumptions about themselves, their patients, and their interactions in the course of medical practice.
>
> (Hahn 1995, 268–69

As Hahn humbly states in his review of the literature on biomedical practice, he is not the first to observe this. However, he is among the first to make a powerful argument for the institutionalization of what he terms "anthropological medicine":

> a theory and practice that gives primacy to sickness—conditions of patients as conceived as unwanted by themselves—that accepts the social and cultural roots of both professional and lay ideas and attitudes of sickness; that fully recognizes the etiology of sickness in social and cultural as well as physiological and environmental conditions; that also acknowledges sociocultural effects in therapy and healing processes and respects the social context of healing. . . . It integrates a sociocultural perspective with a biological one at the core of medical education, medical practice, research, and institutional arrangements.
>
> (Hahn 1995, 265)

In effect, Hahn argues that because medicine is at heart cross-cultural—because patients and healers always bring (at least slightly and sometimes widely) different ideas with them to their clinical

·

encounters—"an anthropological perspective is a basic and essential component of good medical theory and practice rather than a peripheral, optional one" (1995, 266). Listening, understanding sociocultural context, and recognizing intraethnic variability are key principles of medicine in Hahn's view. Good practice also depends on explaining, translating, and brokering between cultural worlds, and respecting, responding, and accommodating others' needs and desires.

Hahn's point about intraethnic variability merits additional comment here. Throughout this book, we have included examples from many cultural and social contexts. We have sometimes drawn attention to syndromes that occur most commonly in specific cultural contexts or that people from given cultures attend to, such as susto, empacho, high blood, and high-pertension. We have done so in an effort to bring some life and immediacy to the theoretical concepts we are attempting to illustrate. However, we have made a complementary effort not to suggest that particular formulas for ethnic or cultural sensitivity be followed in constructing clinical care regimens, but rather to argue that caregivers maintain flexibility and develop cultural assessment skills, so they can take into account patients' individual needs (Hahn 1995; Majumdar 1995).

In all clinical encounters, the cultural models described by patients and evident in the histories given are not an ending point but rather a starting point—a place from which a discussion of what to do next can begin (cf. Kleinman et al. 1978). As Fox reminds us, cultural competence involves more than simply becoming aware of and sensitive to other cultures. Unconscious attitudes and biases still may lie below the surface and influence clinical decision making. It is therefore necessary for health care providers to thoroughly examine their own cultures first and foremost. One's own culture "is far from a neutral background against which other cultures are measured" (2005, 1316).

THE CALL FOR NEW PARADIGMS, OR MULTICULTURALISM REVISITED

There has been much recognition of the need for new or expanded paradigms for the delivery of health and medical care. We argue that any new paradigm *must* consider and include cultural diversity in prevention, diagnosis, and treatment. Science is vital, but its interpretations and applications have become inadequate to meet the challenges faced by the health care system. Ultimate solutions must be located within the human condition, with additional focus on culture, and on individual *and* social responsibility.

The biomedical model, long associated with core U.S. values and superiority, has led to impressive improvements in heath care. However, it is not directed to meet the human challenges wrought by social and technological change. New strategies must be incorporated within the delivery system to meet current needs—strategies focused on links and interrelationships, rather than supremacy of one sector over others.

Race, class, gender, and age supremacy, for instance, although never justified, are today challenged by simple demographics. Providers as well as patients now come from increasingly diverse backgrounds. Women and minorities are moving steadily into the field of medicine. Because of demographic trends, "older adults, including the 'baby boomers,' will be cared for by large numbers of health care professionals who are people of color, and will be financially supported by the taxes of large numbers of younger people of color" (Feagin, Vera, and Zsembik 1996, 17). This is sadly ironic, given present inequities in health care access and outcomes.

The orientation of medicine's service to suffering humanity should not distinguish or select to whom that service will be given. The art of medicine is the art of human relationships and communication, and, most of all, *caring*. But biomedicine is not acultural. It responds in shape to changing needs and expectations as part of an expanding multicultural world. As Feagin and colleagues have noted, many of the so-called ethnic conflicts in the world are generated by the demand for economic, political, and social recognition and power: "The unique identities of individuals can be respected only when each group and culture is fully respected and equally influential. Diversity is thus coterminous with real democracy" (1996, 19). The challenge is there for all of us.

FOR DISCUSSION

1. What barriers to health care are encountered by impoverished minority women? How do these compare to the barriers encountered by impoverished minority men, by recent immigrants, and by gay people? How do these barriers help to create and maintain syndemics?

2. How did modernization and globalization contribute to the spread of AIDS? How does sexism contribute to the spread of AIDS? How does racism contribute?

3. Discuss the impact that the association between AIDS and homosexuality and drug use has had on the public's response to the disease. Identify another disease and likewise analyze the stigmas associated, as well as what their hidden functions might be.

4. Try to identify some of the means and methods of integrating complementary and alternative health care modalities into mainstream health care delivery in the United States. Find examples of resistance as well. To what extent can (or should) integration take place, and how can we bridge the gaps?

5. How can we best promote a multicultural approach to health care, or "sociocultural medicine"? Suggest and discuss some possibilities and innovations.

Appendix A: Project and Class Presentation Ideas

Here are some projects that readers can undertake to further learning or to provide grist for a presentation. The ideas also can provide material for reflecting upon during group discussions or personal perusals at appropriate junctures in the reading.

1. Identify a medical system that is foreign to you and learn all you can about it. Develop a presentation by which you can describe and explain the system to your classmates, systematically comparing and contrasting the system you have chosen to our own (biomedical) system of care, perhaps referring to ideas from Chapter 4.

2. Observe customers in the vitamin or nutritional supplement section of a supermarket or drugstore for two hours (it is a good idea to let the manager know that you are doing a class project). What walks of life did customers come from (and who seemed to be missing)? How did these people seem to handle their selections? What barriers or facilitators did they seem to encounter? How might price or advertising have come into play? What seems to attract people, and what kinds of people are attracted to what sorts of displays?

3. Survey two weeks' worth of newspapers or the equivalent for contagious disease–related stories or stories on changes in health care policy, or technology. Examine these stories for bias. What patterns emerge? How do they relate to cultural understandings or social

processes? (Different groups of students might be assigned to monitor reporting on different specific topics; different groups also might be assigned to monitor different kinds of media, as relevant: radio talk or news shows of diverse origins, various types of magazines, national or local newspapers, tabloids, official government Web sites, etc.)

4. Design a hand-washing promotion intervention for two particular cultural groups in your town, including the cultural group to which you belong. What cultural factors would have to be kept in mind? What socioeconomic, age-related, or gender-linked factors also would need to be considered? Look at other campaigns such as the antismoking campaign. Why was it successful?

5. Conduct a fact-finding mission about medical travel patterns among your classmates or at your school or in your neighborhood or city. Who travels across regional, state, or national borders for health care? What kind of care do they travel for, and why? Are certain subgroups more likely than others to opt for medical travel? Why do you think this is? What do you think should be done (if anything) to regulate cross-border health trade?

6. Select a particular health hazard or risk, for instance one's risk for heart disease or for a particular kind of traumatic injury. Test the strength, in your class or with another group, of the optimistic bias in regard to this risk (see Chapter 8). With the help of your instructor, design a survey to measure how "at risk" people feel. Do they feel that their chances of contracting or suffering from the condition in question are high or low? Why? How do they compare their own risks with those of most of their peers? On what basis is that comparison made? How do you explain this and your other findings?

7. Keep a health care diary for four weeks. Try to record each night anything that happened to you during the day related to health, illness, or care seeking. Did you have a headache? Did you catch a cold? Did you twist your ankle? Did you eat something that disagreed with you? Were you extremely tired or have muscle aches? Anything goes, as long as you notice it. What did you do about it? Why? Put the diary away for a few days and then read it over. What patterns do you notice? How do they relate to your socialization, your gender, your role or socioeconomic status? Note anything that relates to your cultural identity. What lessons can you draw from this exercise?

Appendix B: Relevant Web Sites

1. Cultural competence resources

Agency for Healthcare Research and Quality (AHRQ)—Cultural and Linguistic Competency	http://www.ahrq.gov/path/compath.htm
Center for Communications Programs, Johns Hopkins University	http://www.jhuccp.org
Centers for Disease Control and Prevention (CDC): Life Stages and Specific Populations	http://www.cdc.gov/LifeStages/
Cross-Cultural Healthcare Program	http://www.xculture.org
Diversity RX	http://www.diversityrx.org
EthnoMed	http://ethnomed.org/
Health Resources and Services Administration (HRSA): Cultural Competence Resources	http://www.hrsa.gov/culturalcompetence/
Institute for Diversity in Health Management	http://www.diversityconnection.org

National Center for Cultural Competence, Georgetown University	http://nccc.georgetown.edu/index.html
National Council on Interpreting in Healthcare	http://www.ncihc.org
National Standards on Culturally and Linguistically Appropriate Services (CLAS)	http://raceandhealth.hhs.gov/templates/browse.aspx?lvl=2&lvlID=15
Office of Minority Health (OMH): Cultural Competency Section	http://minorityhealth.hhs.gov/templates/browse.aspx?lvl=1&lvlID=3
Office of Minority Health (OMH): Think Cultural Health / Center for Linguistic and Cultural Competence in Health Care (CLCCHC)	https://www.thinkculturalhealth.org/
Program for Multicultural Health, University of Michigan	http://www.med.umich.edu/Multicultural/ccp/culcomp.htm

2. General resources

Centers for Disease Control and Prevention (CDC)	http://www.cdc.gov
Centers for Disease Control and Prevention (CDC): National Center for Health Statistics	http://www.cdc.gov/nchs
Healthy People 2010	http://www.healthypeople.gov/
National Center for Complementary and Alternative Medicine (NCCAM)	http://nccam.nih.gov/
National Institute of Nursing Research (NINR)	http://www.nih.gov/ninr
National Institutes of Health (NIH)	http://nih.gov
National Women's Health Information Center	http://www.4woman.org
Office for Civil Rights	http://www.dhhs.gov/ocr

| Office of Minority Health | http://minorityhealth.hhs.gov/ |
| World Health Organization | http://www.who.int/ |

3. Professional, academic, and nongovernmental organizations (NGOs)

AcademyHealth	http://www.academyhealth.org/
American Holistic Health Association	http://www.ahha.org
American Medical Association	http://www.ama-assn.org
American Psychological Association	http://www.apa.org
California Nurses Association	www.calnurses.org
Doctors without Borders	http://www.DoctorsWithoutBorders.org
Hastings Center for Bioethics	http://www.thehastingscenter.org
Medical Sociology Section of the American Sociological Association	http://dept.kent.edu/sociology/asamedsoc/
National Association of Social Workers	http://www.socialworkers.org/
Partners in Health	http://www.pih.org
Physicians for a National Health Program	http://pnhp.org
Physicians for Social Responsibility	http://www.psr.org
Transcultural Nursing Society	http://www.tcns.org

Bibliography

Abelove, H. 1994. "The Politics of the 'Gay Plague': AIDS as a U.S. Ideology," in *Body Politics: Disease, Desire, and the Family*. M. Ryan and A. Gordon, eds. 3–17. San Francisco: Westview Press.

Adair, J., K. Deuschle, and C. Barnett. 1988 [1972]. *The People's Health: Anthropology and Medicine in a Navajo Community*, Rev. and expanded ed. Albuquerque: University of New Mexico Press.

Adams, P., and V. Benson. 1991. "Current Estimates from the National Health Interview Survey, 1990." National Center for Health Statistics. *Vital Health Statistics* 10: 181.

AIDS Alert. 1993. "Research Gaining Support for Vaginal Microbicide." 8(9): 134.

American College of Physicians. 2006. *The Advanced Medical Home: A Patient-Centered, Physician-Guided Model of Health Care*. Policy monograph. Philadelphia: American College of Physicians.

Anderson, E. 1990. *Streetwise: Race, Class, and Change in an Urban Neighborhood*. Chicago: University of Chicago Press.

Annas, G. 1994. "Women, Health Care, and the Law: Birth, Death, and In Between," in *An Unfinished Revolution: Women and Health Care in America*. E. Friedman, ed. 29–45. New York: United Hospital Fund of New York.

Arber, S., and H. Thomas. 2005. "From Women's Health to a Gender Analysis of Health," in *The Blackwell Companion to Medical Sociology*. W. Cockerham, ed. 94–113. Oxford: Blackwell.

Archibold, R. C. 2008. "Indians' Water Rights Give Hope for Better Health." *New York Times*, August 30, national edition, sec. 1.

As noted in the Preface, the bibliography has been updated to reflect new developments *except* where new scholarship simply corroborates older observations. Therefore, a certain number of older references have been retained in the present bibliographic list.

Arellano, R., and S. Kearny. 1992. *Cultural Considerations (A Supplement to Teaching Hospital: Cultural Determinants of Health and Illness and Their Importance in Effective Health- Care Delivery at University Hospital)*. Albuquerque: Creative Services/ Dissemination Unit of the Health of the Public Program, University of New Mexico School of Medicine.

Aries, P. 1974. *Western Attitudes Toward Death: From the Middle Ages to the Present*. Baltimore: Johns Hopkins University Press.

Armstrong, D. 1987. "Theoretical Tensions in Biopsychosocial Medicine." *Social Science and Medicine* 25(11): 1213–18.

———. 1989. *An Outline of Sociology as Applied to Medicine*, 3rd ed. London: Wright.

Atchley, R. 1994. *Social Forces and Aging: An Introduction to Social Gerontology*, 7th ed. Belmont, CA: Wadsworth.

Augé, M., and C. Herzlich, eds. 1995 [1983]. *The Meaning of Illness: Anthropology, History and Sociology*. Translated from the French by K. Durnin, C. Lambein, K. Leclercq-Jones, B. Garnier, and R. Williams. London: Harwood Academic.

Baer, H. 1989. "The American Dominative Medical System as a Reflection of Social Relations in the Larger Society." *Social Science and Medicine* 28(11): 1103–12.

———. 2001. *Biomedicine and Alternative Healing Systems in America*. Madison: University of Wisconsin Press.

Baer, H., M. Singer, and J. Johnsen. 1986. "Toward a Critical Medical Anthropology." *Social Science and Medicine* 23(2): 95–98.

Baer, R. 1996. "Health and Mental Health Among Mexican-Americans: Implications for Survey Research." *Human Organization* 55(1): 58–66.

Bailey, R. C., and S. D. Mehta. 2009. "Circumcision's Place in the Vicious Cycle Involving Herpes Simplex Virus Type 2 and HIV." *Journal of Infectious Diseases* 199: 923–25.

Baker, L., T. Wagner, S. Singer, and M. Bundorff. 2003. "Use of the Internet and E-mail for Health Care Information Results from a National Survey." *Journal of the American Medical Association* 289: 2400–2406.

Barker, K. 2008. "Electronic Support Groups, Patient-Consumers, and Medicalization: The Case of Contested Illness." *Journal of Health and Social Behavior* 49: 20–38.

Barnes, B. 1985. *About Science*. New York: Basil Blackwell.

Barnes, P. M., B. Bloom, and R. L. Nahin. 2008. "Complementary and Alternative Medicine Use Among Adults and Children: United States, 2007." National Health Statistics Reports; no 12. Hyattsville, MD: National Center for Health Statistics.

Barr, D. 2008. *Health Disparities in the United States: Social Class, Race, Ethnicity, and Health*. Baltimore: Johns Hopkins University Press.

Bart, P. 1969. *Why Women's Status Changes with Middle Age*. Sociological Symposium, no. 3. Blacksburg: Virginia Polytechnic Institute and State University, Department of Sociology.

Bashshur, R., T. Reardon, and G. Shannon. 2000. "Telemedicine: A New Health Care Delivery System." *Annual Review of Public Health* 21(1): 613–37 (doi:10.1146/ annurev.publhealth.21.1.613).

Bayer, R., and A. L. Fairchild. 2006. "Changing the Paradigm for HIV Testing: The End of Exceptionalism." *New England Journal of Medicine* 355(7): 647–49.

Becker, A. 1994. "Nurturing and Negligence: Working on Others' Bodies in Fiji," in *Embodiment and Experience: The Existential Ground of Culture and Self.* T. Csordas, ed. 100–115. Cambridge: Cambridge University Press.

Becker, M., ed. 1974. *The Health Belief Model and Personal Health Behavior.* San Francisco: Society for Public Health Education.

Becker, M., and L. Maiman. 1975. *The Health Belief Model and Personal Health Behavior.* San Francisco: Society for Public Health Education.

Beckford, J. 1984. "Holistic Imagery and Ethics in New Religious and Healing Movements." *Social Compass* 21(2–3): 259–72.

Beckman, H., K. Markakis, A. Suchman, and R. Frankel. 1994. "The Doctor-Patient Relationship and Malpractice: Lessons from Plaintiff Depositions." *Archives of Internal Medicine* 154: 1365–70.

Behrhorst, C. 1993. "The Chimaltenango Development Program," in *A New Dawn in Guatemala: Toward a Worldwide Health Vision.* R. Luecke, ed. 55–76. Prospect Heights, IL: Waveland Press.

Benson, H., with M. Klipper. 2000. *The Relaxation Response.* New York: Avon Books.

Bente, G., M. Senokozlieva, S. Pennig, A. Al-Issa, A., and O. Fischer. (2008). "Deciphering the Secret Code: A New Methodology for the Cross-Cultural Analysis of Nonverbal Behavior." *Behavior Research Methods* 40(1), 269–77.

Berkow, R., ed. 1982. *Merck Manual of Diagnosis and Therapy.* Rahway, NJ: Merck Sharp & Dohme Research Laboratories.

Berliner, H. 1975. "A Larger Perspective on the Flexner Report." *International Journal of Health Services* 5(4): 573–92.

Berliner, H., and J. Salmon. 1980. "The Holistic Alternative to Scientific Medicine: History and Analysis." *International Journal of Health Services* 10(1): 133–47.

Bernard, H. 2001. *Research Methods in Anthropology: Qualitative and Quantitative Approaches,* 3rd ed. Walnut Creek, CA: AltaMira Press.

Bettelheim, B. 1962 [1954]. *Symbolic Wounds: Puberty Rites and the Envious Male.* New York: Collier Books.

Bezemer, W. 1992. "Women and HIV." *Journal of Psychology and Human Sexuality* 5(1,2): 31–36.

Bhatia, J., D. Vir, A. Timmappaya, and C. Chuttani. 1975. "Traditional Healers and Modern Medicine." *Social Science and Medicine* 9(1): 15–21.

Bigby, J., ed. 2003. *Cross-Cultural Medicine.* Philadelphia: American College of Physicians.

Bird, C., and P. Rieker. 2008. *Gender and Health: The Effects of Constrained Choices: and Social Policies.* New York: Cambridge University Press.

Bird, C., P. Conrad, and A. Fremont, eds. 2000. *Handbook of Medical Sociology,* 5th ed. Upper Saddle River, NJ: Prentice Hall.

Bishop, T. F., and N. Kathuria. (2008). "Economic and Healthcare Forces of Hospitalist Movement." *Mount Sinai Journal of Medicine* 75(5): 424–29.

Bletzer, K. 1993. "Migrant HIV Education in the Wake of the AIDS Crisis." *Practicing Anthropology* 15(4): 13–16.

Blumenthal, R. 1988. "10 Are Indicted in Major Fraud on Blood Tests." *New York Times,* New York edition, sec. 1.

Bodeker, G. 1996. "Global Health Traditions," in *Fundamentals of Complementary and Alternative Medicine*. M. Micozzi, ed. 279–90. New York: Churchill Livingstone.

Bollini, P., and H. Siem. 1995. "No Real Progress Towards Equity: Health of Migrants and Ethnic Minorities on the Eve of the Year 2000." *Social Science and Medicine* 41(6): 819–28.

Bolton, R. 1992. "AIDS and Promiscuity: Muddles in the Models," in *Rethinking AIDS Prevention*. R. Bolton and M. Singer, eds. 7–85. New York: Gordon and Breach Science.

Bolton, R., and M. Singer. 1992. "Introduction. Rethinking HIV Prevention: Critical Assessments of the Content and Delivery of AIDS Risk-Reduction Messages," in *Rethinking AIDS Prevention*. R. Bolton and M. Singer, eds. 1–5. New York: Gordon and Breach Science.

Bookman, M. Z., and K. R. Bookman. (2007). *Medical Tourism in Developing Countries*. New York: Palgrave Macmillan.

Borden, W. 1991. "Beneficial Outcomes in Adjustment to HIV Seropositivity." *Social Service Review* 65(3): 434–49.

Bordo, S. 1993. *Unbearable Weight: Feminism, Western Culture, and the Body*. Los Angeles: University of California Press.

Boston Women's Health Book Collective. 1973. *Our Bodies, Ourselves: A Book by and for Women*. New York: Simon and Schuster.

Boulis, A., and J. Jacobs. 2008. *The Changing Face of Medicine: Women Doctors and the Evolution of Health Care in America*. Ithaca, NY: Cornell University Press.

Brach, C., and I. Fraser. 2000. "Can Cultural Competency Reduce Racial and Ethnic Disparities? A Review and Conceptual Model." *Medical Care Research and Review* 57(Suppl. 1): 181–217.

Brandt, A. 1991. "Emerging Themes in the History of Medicine." *The Milbank Quarterly* 69(2): 199–214.

Brink, P. J. 1989. "The Fattening Room among the Annang of Nigeria." *Medical Anthropology* 12: 131–43.

Broverman, J., D. Broverman, F., Clarkson, P., Rosenkrantz, and S. Vogel. 1970. "Sex Role Stereotypes and Clinical Judgments of Mental Health." *Journal of Consulting and Clinical Psychiatry* 34(1): 1–7.

Brown, E. 1979. *Rockefeller Medicine Men*. Berkeley: University of California Press.

Brown, P. 1995. "Naming and Framing: The Social Construction of Diagnosis and Illness." *Journal of Health and Social Behavior* (Extra issue): 34–52.

Brownstein, J., C. Freifeld, and L. Madoff. 2009. "Digital Disease Detection—Harnessing the Web for Public Health Surveillance." http://www.nejm.org (10.1056/NEJMp0900702).

Burton, J. W. (2001). *Culture and the Human Body*. Long Grove, IL: Waveland Press.

Bury, M., and J. Gabe, eds. 2004. *The Sociology of Health and Illness: A Reader*. New York: Routledge.

California Newsreel. 2008a. *Finding Hope for the Future by Reclaiming the Past*. San Francisco: California Newsreel.

———. 2008b. *Unnatural Causes: When the Bough Breaks*. San Francisco: California Newsreel with Vital Pictures, Inc.

———. 2008c. *Unnatural Causes: In Sickness and in Wealth*. San Francisco: California Newsreel with Vital Pictures, Inc.

Cameron, C. 1996. "Patient Compliance: Recognition of Factors Involved and Suggestions for Promoting Compliance with Therapeutic Regimens." *Journal of Advanced Nursing* 24(2): 244–50.

Campbell, C. 1990. "Women and AIDS." *Social Science and Medicine* 30(4): 407–15.

Cassell, J. 1998. *The Woman in the Surgeon's Body*. Cambridge, MA: Harvard University Press.

Cassidy, C. 1991. "The Good Body: When Bigger Is Better." *Medical Anthropology* 13: 181–213.

Cassileth, B., E. Lusk, T. Strouse, and B. Bodenheimer. 1884. "Contemporary Unorthodox Treatments in Cancer Medicine: A Study of Patients, Treatments, and Practitioners." *Annals of Internal Medicine* 101: 105–12.

Centers for Disease Control and Prevention. 1993a. *HIV/AIDS Prevention* 4(2). Atlanta: Centers for Disease Control and Prevention.

———. 1993b. *HIV/AIDS Surveillance Report* 5(2). Atlanta: Centers for Disease Control and Prevention.

———. 1995. *HIV/AIDS Surveillance Report* 7(2). Atlanta: Centers for Disease Control and Prevention.

———. 2002. "Hysterectomy Surveillance—United States, 1994–1999." http:www.cdc.gov/mmwr/preview/mmwrhtml/ss5105a1.htm (accessed November 18, 2009).

———. 2006. "Youth Risk Behavior Surveillance—United States, 2005." *Surveillance Summaries, Morbidity and Mortality Weekly Report* 55(SS-5). Atlanta: Centers for Disease Control and Prevention.

———. 2008a. "CDC HIV/AIDS Fact Sheet: HIV/AIDS Among Women." Atlanta: Centers for Disease Control and Prevention.

———. 2009a. *HIV/AIDS Surveillance Report, Volume 19: Cases of HIV Infection and AIDS in the United States and Dependent Areas, 2007*. Atlanta: Department of Health and Human Services, Centers for Disease Control and Prevention.

———. 2009b. Injury—A Risk at Any Stage of Life. In *CDC Injury Fact Book*. CDC, ed. 31–34. Atlanta: Centers for Disease Control and Prevention.

Centers for Disease Control and Prevention and National Center for Chronic Disease Prevention and Health Promotion. 2009. *Injury & Violence (Including Suicide)*. Atlanta: Centers for Disease Control and Prevention.

Centers for Disease Control and Prevention/National Center for Health Statistics. 2009. *Fast Stats: Infant Death*. Atlanta: Centers for Disease Control and Prevention, Office of Information Services.

CensusScope. n.d. *United States: Household and Family Structure*. Social Science Data Analysis Network. http://www.censusscope.org/us/chart_house.html.

Chadwick, B., and T. Heaton, eds. 1992. *Statistical Handbook on the American Family*. New York: Oryx Press.

Chen, A., and W. Rogan. 2004. "Breastfeeding and the Risk of Postneonatal Death in the United States." *Pediatrics* 113(5): e435–e39.

Cheng, T., J. Savageua, A. Sattler, and T. DeWitt. 1993. "Confidentiality in Health Care: A Survey of Knowledge, Perceptions, and Attitudes among High School Students." *Journal of the American Medical Association* 269(11): 1404–7.

Chrisman, N. 1977. "The Health Seeking Process: An Approach to the Natural History of Illness." *Culture, Medicine and Psychiatry* 1: 351–77.

Clark, J., D. Potter, and J. McKinlay. 1991. "Bringing Social Structure Back into Clinical Decision Making." *Social Science and Medicine* 8: 853–66.

Clements, F. 1932. "Primitive Concepts of Disease." *University of California Publications in American Archaeology and Ethnology* 32: 185–252.

Cochran, S. 1989. "Women and HIV Infection: Issues in Prevention and Behavioral Change," in *Primary Prevention of AIDS: Psychological Approaches*. V. Mays, G. Albee, and S. Schneider, eds. 309–27. Newbury Park, CA: Sage.

Cockerham, W. 1995. *Medical Sociology*, 6th ed. Englewood Cliffs, NJ: Prentice Hall.

———. 2000. "The Sociology of Health Behavior and Health Lifestyles," in *Handbook of Medical Sociology*, 5th ed. C. Bird, P. Conrad, and A. Fremont, eds. 159–72. Upper Saddle River, NJ: Prentice Hall.

———., ed. 2005. *The Blackwell Companion to Medical Sociology*. Oxford: Blackwell.

———. 2010. *Medical Sociology*, 11th ed. Upper Saddle River, NJ: Prentice Hall.

Coe, R. 1978. *Sociology of Medicine*, 2nd ed. New York: McGraw- Hill.

Coney, S. 1994. *The Menopause Industry: How the Medical Establishment Exploits Women*, U.S. ed., rev. Alameda, CA: Hunter House.

Conover, K. 1993. "Trucking Through the AIDS Belt." *New Yorker*, August 16, 56 ff.

Conrad, P. 2000. "Medicalization, Genetics, and Human Problems," in *Handbook of Medical Sociology*, 5th ed. C. Bird and A. Fremont, eds. 322–33. Upper Saddle River, NJ: Prentice Hall.

———. 2007. *The Medicalization of Society: On the Transformation of Human Conditions into Treatable Disorders*. Baltimore: Johns Hopkins University Press.

Conrad, P., and J. Schneider. 1992. *Deviance and Medicalization: From Badness to Sickness*, Expanded ed. Philadelphia: Temple University Press.

Cook, R. 1972. *The Year of the Intern*. New York: The New American Library.

Corea, G. 1977. *The Hidden Malpractice: How American Medicine Mistreats Women*. New York: Jove/HBJ.

Corr, C., C. Nabe, and D. Corr. 1997. *Death and Dying: Life and Living*, 2nd ed. Pacific Grove, CA: Brooks/Cole.

Cousins, N. 1979. *Anatomy of an Illness*. New York: Norton.

———. 1981 [1979]. *Anatomy of an Illness as Perceived by the Patient: Reflections on Healing and Regeneration*. New York: Bantam Books.

Cowgill, D. 1972. *Aging and Modernization*. New York: Appleton-Century-Crofts.

Crosson, F. J. 2005. "The Delivery System Matters." *Health Affairs* 24(6): 1543–48.

Darkins, A., and M. Cary. 2000. *Telemedicine and Telehealth: Principles, Policies, Performance, and Pitfalls*. New York: Springer.

Davis, D., and R. Whitten. 1987. "The Cross-Cultural Study of Human Sexuality." *Annual Reviews in Anthropology* 16: 69–98.

Davis-Floyd, R. 1992. *Birth as an American Rite of Passage*. Los Angeles: University of California Press.

———. 2003. *Birth as an American Rite of Passage*, 2nd ed. Los Angeles: University of California Press.

De, D., and J. Richardson. 2008. "Cultural Safety: An Introduction." *Paediatric Nursing* 20(2): 39–43.

Demakis, J. G., C. Beauchamp, W. L. Cull, R. Denwood, S. A. Eisen, R. Lofgren, K. Nichol, J. Woolliscroft, and W. G. Henderson. (2000). "Improving Residents' Compliance with Standards of Ambulatory Care: Results from the VA

Cooperative Study on Computerized Reminders." *Journal of the American Medical Association* 284(11): 1411–16.

Demers, R., R. Altamore, H. Mustin, A. Kleinman, and D. Leonardi. 1980. "An Exploration of the Dimensions of Illness Behavior." *Journal of Family Practice* 11: 1085–92.

DeParle, J. 1990. "Talk of Government Being Out to Get Blacks Falls on More Attentive Ears," *New York Times*, October 29, sec. 2.

Dietz, T. 1995. "Patterns of Intergenerational Assistance within the Mexican-American Family: Is the Family Taking Care of the Older Generations' Needs?" *Journal of Family Issues* 16(3): 344–56.

DiMatteo, M., and D. DiNicola. 1982. *Achieving Patient Compliance: The Psychology of the Medical Practitioner's Role*. New York: Pergamon Press.

Dominguez, T. (2008). "Race, Racism, and Racial Disparities in Adverse Birth Outcomes." *Clinical Obstetrics and Gynecology* 51(2): 360–70.

Dossey, L. 1982. *Space, Time and Medicine*. Boulder, CO: Shambhala.

———. 1991. *Meaning and Medicine*. New York: Bantam Books.

Dow, J. 1986. "Universal Aspects of Symbolic Meaning: A Theoretical Synthesis." *American Anthropologist* 88(1): 56–69.

Dowling, M. 2009. "N.J. Corruption Probe Includes First Organ Trafficking Case." *The Star-Ledger*, July 24.

Data Resource Center for Child and Adolescent Health. 2009. *Who Are Children with Special Health Care Needs?* Portland: Child and Adolescent Health Measurement Initiative at Oregon Health & Science University.

Dressler, W. 1990. "Culture, Stress and Disease," in *Medical Anthropology: Contemporary Theory and Method*. T. Johnson and C. Sargent, eds. 248–67. New York: Praeger.

Durose, M.R., C. W. Harlow, P. A. Langan, M. Motivans, R. R. Rantala, and E. L. Schmitt. 2005. "Family Violence Statistics: Including Statistics on Strangers and Acquaintances" (NCJ 207846). Washington, DC: Bureau of Justice Statistics. http://bjs.ojp.usdoj.gov/index.cfm?ty=pbdetail&iid=828.

Dutton, D. 1978. "Explaining the Low Use of Health Services by the Poor: Costs, Attitudes, or Delivery Systems?" *American Sociological Review* 43(June): 348–68.

Eagan, A. 1994. "The Women's Health Movement and Its Lasting Impact," in *An Unfinished Revolution: Health Care in America*. E. Friedman, ed. 15–27. New York: United Hospital Fund of New York.

Eastman, K., and M. Loustaunau. 1987. "Reacting to the Medical Bureaucracy: Lay Midwifery as a Birthing Alternative." *Marriage and Family Review* 11(3–4): 23–37.

Economist. 2001. "At Last, Good News on the Family (Probably)." July 28, 29–30.

———. 2008a. "Importing Competition." Globalisation and Health Care, 388(8593).

———. 2008b. "Operating Profit." Globalisation and Health Care, 388(8593)

———. 2009. "I Am Just a Poor Boy Though My Story's Seldom Told." Neuroscience and Social Deprivation, 391(8625), 82.

Edgar, H. 1992. "Outside the Community." *Hastings Center Report* 22(6): 32–35.

Eisenberg, D., R. Kessler, C. Foster, F. Norlock, D. Calkins, and T. Delbanco. 1993. "Unconventional Medicine in the United States: Prevalence, Costs, and Patterns of Use." *New England Journal of Medicine* 328(4): 246–52.

Eisenberg, L., and A. Kleinman, eds. 1985. *The Relevance of Social Science for Medicine*. Dordrecht, Netherlands: D. Reidel.

Eisenbruch, M. 1984. "Cross-Cultural Aspects of Bereavement. II: Ethnic and Cultural Variations in the Development of Bereavement Practices." *Culture, Medicine and Psychiatry* 8: 315–47.

Emanuel, E., and L. Emanuel. 1992. "Four Models of the Physician-Patient Relationship." *Journal of the American Medical Association* 267(16): 2221–26.

Engel, G. 1977. "The Need for a New Medical Model: A Challenge for Biomedicine." *Science* 196: 129–36.

Ergil, K. 1996. "China's Traditional Medicine," in *Fundamentals of Complementary and Alternative Medicine*. M. Micozzi, ed. 185–230. New York: Churchill Livingstone.

Etkin, N. 1990. "Ethnopharmacology: Biological and Behavioral Perspectives in the Study of Indigenous Medicines," in *Medical Anthropology: Contemporary Theory and Method*. T. Johnson and C. Sargent, eds. 149–58. New York: Praeger.

Fagin, C. 1994. "Women and Nursing: A Historical Perspective," in *An Unfinished Revolution: Women and Health Care in America*. E. Friedman, ed. 159–76. New York: United Hospital Fund of New York.

Farmer, P. (2001). *AIDS and Accusation: Haiti and the Geography of Blame*. Los Angeles: University of California Press.

———. (1999). *Infections and Inequalities: The Modern Plagues*. Los Angeles: University of California Press.

———. (2005). *Pathologies of Power: Health, Human Rights, and the New War on the Poor*. Los Angeles: University of California Press.

Feagin, J., H. Vera, and B. Zsembik. 1996. "Multiculturalism: A Democratic Basis for U.S. Society," in *Perspectives on Sociology*. C. Calhoun and G. Ritzer, eds. 1–22. New York: McGraw-Hill.

Fee, E. 1989. "Henry E. Sigerist: From the Social Production of Disease to Medical Management and Scientific Socialism." *Milbank Quarterly* 67(Suppl. 1): 127–50.

Ferraro, G., W. Trevathan, and J. Levy. 1994. *Anthropology: An Applied Perspective*. San Francisco: West.

Fischoff, B., S. Lichtenstein, P. Slovic, S. L. Derby, and R. L. Keeny. 1981. *Acceptable Risk*. New York: Cambridge University Press.

Fisher, E. 2008. "Building a Medical Neighborhood for the Medical Home." *New England Journal of Medicine* 359(12): 1202–5.

Flexner, A. 1910. *Medical Education in the United States and Canada: A Report to the Carnegie Foundation for the Advancement of Teaching*, Bulletin 4. Boston: D. B. Updike, Merrymount Press.

Flint, M. 1975. "The Menopause: Reward or Punishment?" *Psychosomatics* 16: 161–63.

Ford, V. 2009. "Nursing Perspectives in Addressing Health Disparities," in *Cultural Proficiency in Addressing Health Disparities*. S. Kosoko-Lasaki, C. Cook, and R. O'Brien, eds. 87–98. Sudbury, MA: Jones and Bartlett.

Forster, H., J. Schwartz, and E. DeRenzo. 2002. "Reducing Legal Risk by Practicing Patient-centered Medicine." *Archives of Internal Medicine* 162(11): 1217–19.

Foster, G. 1976. "Disease Etiologies in Non-Western Medical Systems." *American Anthropologist* 78: 773–82.

———. 1978. "Medical Anthropology: Some Contrasts with Medical Sociology," in *Health and the Human Condition: Perspectives on Medical Anthropology*. M. Logan and E. Hunt Jr., eds. 2–11. North Scituate, MA: Duxbury Press.

———. 1994. *Hippocrates' Latin American Legacy: Humoral Medicine in the New World*. Amsterdam: Gordon and Breach.

Foucault, M. 1975 [1963]. *The Birth of the Clinic*. New York: Vintage.

Fox, R. 1977. "The Medicalization and Demedicalization of American Society." *Daedalus* 106(9): 9–22.

———. 1989. *The Sociology of Medicine: A Participant Observer's View*. Englewood Cliffs, NJ: Prentice Hall.

———. 1994. "The Entry of U.S. Bioethics into the 1990s," in *A Matter of Principles?: Ferment in U.S. Bioethics*. E. DuBose, R. Hamel, and L. O'Connell, eds. 21–71. Valley Forge, PA: Trinity Press International.

———. 2005. "Cultural Competence and the Culture of Medicine." *New England Journal of Medicine* 353: 1316–17.

Frankenberg, R. 1994. "The Impact of HIV/AIDS on Concepts Relating to Risk and Culture Within British Community Epidemiology: Candidates or Targets for Prevention." *Social Science and Medicine* 18(10): 1325–35.

Fraser, S., ed. 1995. *The Bell Curve Wars: Race, Intelligence, and the Future of America*. New York: Basic Books.

Frazer, J. 1942 [1922]. *The Golden Bough: A Study in Magic and Religion*, Abridged ed. New York: Macmillan.

Frazier, H., and F. Mosteller, eds. 1995. *Medicine Worth Paying For*. Cambridge, MA: Harvard University Press.

Freeman, H., R. Blendon, L. Aiken, S. Sudman, C. Mullinix, and C. Corey. 1990. "Americans Report on Their Access to Health Care," in *The Nation's Health*, 3rd ed. P. Lee and C. Estes, eds. 309–19. Boston: Jones and Bartlett.

Freidson, E. 1960. "Client Control and Medical Practice." *American Journal of Sociology* 65:374–82.

———. 1970. *Profession of Medicine: A Study of the Sociology of Applied Knowledge*. New York: Harper and Row.

Freund, P., and M. McGuire. 1995. *Health, Illness, and the Social Body: A Critical Sociology*, 2nd ed. Englewood Cliffs, NJ: Prentice Hall.

Friedman, E. 1994. "Women and Health Care: The Bramble and the Rose," in *An Unfinished Revolution: Women and Health Care in America*. E. Friedman, ed. 1–12. New York: United Hospital Fund of New York.

Fuller, J., and P. Toon. 1988. *Medical Practice in a Multicultural Society*. London: Heinemann.

Funkhouser, S., and D. Moser. 1990. "Is Health Care Racist?" *Advanced Nursing Science* 12(2): 47–55.

Furnham, A., and R. Beard. 1995. "Health, Just World Beliefs and Coping Style Preferences in Patients of Complementary and Orthodox Medicine." *Social Science and Medicine* 40(10): 1425–32.

Galanti, G. 1991. *Caring for Patients from Different Cultures: Case Studies from American Hospitals*. Philadelphia: University of Pennsylvania Press.

———. 2008. *Caring for Patients from Different Cultures: Case Studies from American Hospitals*, 4th ed. Philadelphia: University of Pennsylvania Press.

Gallagher, E., and J. Subedi. 1995. *Global Perspectives on Health Care*. Englewood Cliffs, NJ: Prentice Hall.

Galtung, J. 1969. "Violence, Peace, and Peace Research." *Journal of Peace Research* 6(3): 167–91.

Gardenswartz, L., and A. Rowe. 1998. *Managing Diversity in Health Care*. San Francisco: Jossey-Bass.

Garrett, L. 1994. *The Coming Plague*. New York: Farrar, Straus and Giroux.

Gatter, P. 1995. "Anthropology, HIV and Contingent Identities." *Social Science and Medicine* 41(11): 1523–33.

Gayford, J. 1994. "Domestic Violence," in *Violence in Health Care: A Practical Guide to Coping with Violence and Caring for Victims*. J. Shepherd, ed. 117–34. New York: Oxford University Press.

Gerhardt, U. 1989. *Ideas about Illness*. New York: New York University Press.

Gerth, H., and C. Mills, eds. 1958. *From Max Weber: Essays in Sociology*. New York: Galaxy.

Gesler, W. 1991. *The Cultural Geography of Health Care*. Pittsburgh: University of Pittsburgh Press.

Gillman, M. 2005. "Developmental Origins of Health and Disease." *New England Journal of Medicine* 353(17): 1848–50.

Ginzberg, E. 1990. *The Medical Triangle: Physicians, Politicians, and the Public*. Cambridge, MA: Harvard University Press.

Glass, R. 1996. "The Patient-Physician Relationship: *JAMA* Focuses on the Center of Medicine." *Journal of the American Medical Association* 275(2): 147–48 .

Glazer, N. 1994. "Multiculturalism and Public Policy," in *Values and Public Policy*. H. Aaron, T. Mann, and T. Taylor, eds. 113–45. Washington, DC: Brookings Institution Press.

Global Health Initiative. 2008. "Why Global Health Matters—Here and Abroad." FamiliesUSA: Washington, DC. http://www.familiesusa.org/issues/global -health/matters.

Goffman, E. 1959. *The Presentation of Self in Everyday Life*. New York: Doubleday.

Goldstein, M. 2000. "The Growing Acceptance of Complementary and Alternative Medicine," in *Handbook of Medical Sociology*, 5th ed. C. Bird and A. Fremont, eds. 284–97. Upper Saddle River, NJ: Prentice Hall.

Good, B. 1994. *Medicine, Rationality, and Experience: An Anthropological Perspective*. Cambridge: Cambridge University Press.

Good, B., and M. Delvecchio Good. 1993. " 'Learning Medicine': The Constructing of Medical Knowledge at Harvard Medical School," in *Knowledge, Power and Practice*. S. Lindenbaum and M. Lock, eds. 81–107. Los Angeles: University of California Press.

Gordon, D. 1991. "Female Circumcision and Genital Operations in Egypt and the Sudan: A Dilemma for Medical Anthropology." *Medical Anthropology Quarterly* 5(1): 3–14.

Gordon, G. 1966. *Role Theory and Illness*. New Haven, CT: College and University Press.

Gregor, T. 1985. *Anxious Pleasures*. Chicago: University of Chicago Press.

Groce, N., and I. Zola. 1993. "Multiculturalism, Chronic Illness, and Disability." *Pediatrics* 91(5): 1048–55.

Gross, D. 1992. *Discovering Anthropology*. Mountain View, CA: Mayfield.

Gudykunst, W., ed. 2003. *Cross-Cultural and Intercultural Communication*. Thousand Oaks, CA: Sage.

Gust, D. A., Darling, N., Kennedy, A., and Schwartz, B. (2008). "Parents with Doubts about Vaccines: Which Vaccines and Reasons Why." *Pediatrics* 122: 718–25.

Gustafson, J. 1990. "Moral Discourse About Medicine: A Variety of Forms." *Journal of Medicine and Philosophy* 15: 125–42.

Hafferty, F., and D. Light. 1995. "Professional Dynamics and the Changing Nature of Medical Work." *Journal of Health and Social Behavior* 36(extra issue): 132–53.

Hafferty, F., and J. McKinlay, eds. 1993. *The Changing Medical Profession: An International Perspective*. New York: Oxford University Press.

Hagedorn, H., M. Hogan, J. L. Smith, C. Bowman, G. M. Curran, D. Espadas, B. Kimmel, L. K. Kochevar, M. W. Legro, and A. E. Sales. 2006. "Lessons Learned about Implementing Research Evidence into Clinical Practice: Experiences from VA QUERI." *Journal of General Internal Medicine* (Suppl. 2): S21–24.

Hahn, R. 1984. "Rethinking 'Illness' and 'Disease.'" *Contributions to Asian Studies* 18: 1–23.

———. 1995. *Sickness and Healing: An Anthropological Perspective*. New Haven, CT: Yale University Press.

Hallowell, A. 1977 [1941]. "The Social Function of Anxiety in a Primitive Society," in *Culture, Disease, and Healing: Studies in Medical Anthropology*. D. Landy, ed. 132–38. New York: Macmillan.

Hansen, W., G. Hahn, and B. Wolkenstein. 1990. "Perceived Personal Immunity: Beliefs about Susceptibility to AIDS." *Journal of Sex Research* 27(4): 622–28.

Harper, S., J. Lynch, S. Burris, G. D. Smith. 2007. "Trends in the Black-White Life Expectancy Gap in the United States, 1983–2003." *Journal of the American Medical Association* 297(11): 1224–32.

Harries, A. D., E. J. Schouten, and E. Libamba. 2006. "Scaling Up Antiretroviral Treatment in Resource-Poor Settings." *Lancet* 367: 1870–72.

Hays, R., L. McKusick, L. Pollack, R. Hillard, C. Hoff, and T. Coates. 1993. "Disclosing HIV Seropositivity to Significant Others." *AIDS* 7(3): 425–31.

Health, P. I. (2009). *The PIH Vision: Whatever It Takes*. http://www.pih.org/who/vision.html.

Hechinger, F. 1992. "Adolescent Health: A Generation at Risk." *Carnegie Quarterly* 37(4): 2–16.

Helman, C. 1990. *Culture, Health and Illness*, 2nd ed. Oxford: Butterworth Heinemann.

———. 1995. *Culture, Health and Illness*, 3rd ed. London: Butterworth-Heinemann.

———. (2007). *Culture, Health and Illness*, 5th ed. Oxford: Butterworth-Heinemann

Henry J. Kaiser Family Foundation. 2007. *HIV/AIDS Policy Fact Sheet: The HIV/AIDS Epidemic in the United States*. Menlo Park, CA: Henry J. Kaiser Family Foundation.

———. 2009. "The HIV/AIDS Epidemic in the United States." *HIV/AIDS Policy Fact Sheet* (September). Menlo Park, CA: Henry J. Kaiser Family Foundation. http://www.kff.org/hivaids/upload/3029-10.pdf.

Henslin, J. 2007. *Sociology: A Down-to-Earth Approach*, 8th ed. Boston: Pearson.

Herek, G., and J. Capitanio. 1994. "Conspiracies, Contagion, and Compassion: Trust and Public Reactions to AIDS." *AIDS Education and Prevention* 6(4): 365–75.

Harrell, I. 1992a. "Ethnic Minorities and Health Care: Issues and Solutions." Transcript of talk, Albuquerque, NM.

———. 1992b. *Transcript of Talk on "Ethnic Minorities and Health Care: Issues and Solutions."* Albuquerque, NM: New Mexico.

Hertzman, C., J. Frank, and R. Evans. 1994. "Heterogeneities in Health Status and the Determinants of Population and Health," in *Why Are Some People Healthy and Others Not?: The Determinants of Health of Populations*. R. Evans, M. Barer, and T. Marmor, eds. 67–92. New York: Aldine de Gruyter.

Heurtin-Roberts, S., and E. Reisin. 1990. "Folk Models of Hypertension among Black Women: Problems in Illness Management," in *Anthropology and Primary Health Care*. J. Coreil and D. Mull, eds. 222–50. Boulder, CO: Westview Press.

Hewer, N., G. Boschma, and W. A. Hall. 2009. "Elective Caesarean Section as a Transformative Technological Process: Players, Power and Context." *Journal of Advanced Nursing* 65(8): 1762–71.

Higgins, L. A. (2007). "Medical Tourism Takes Off, But Not without Debate." *Managed Care* 16(4): 45–47.

Hingson, R., and L. Strunin. 1992. "Monitoring Adolescents' Response to the AIDS Epidemic: Changes in Knowledge, Attitudes, Beliefs, and Behaviors," in *Adolescents and AIDS: A Generation in Jeopardy*. R. DiClemente, ed. 3–16. Newbury Park, CA: Sage.

Hollingsworth, J. 1981. "Inequality in Levels of Health in England and Wales, 1891–1971." *Journal of Health and Social Behavior* 22: 268–83.

Holmes, O. 1888. "Currents and Counter-Currents in Medical Science," in *Medical Essays, 1842–1882*. Boston: Houghton Mifflin.

Holmes, T., and R. Rahe. 1967. "The Social Readjustment Rating Scale." *Journal of Psychosomatic Research* 11: 213–18.

Holohan, A. 1977. "Diagnosis: The End of Transition," in *Medical Encounters: The Experience of Illness and Treatment*. A. Davis and G. Horobin, eds. 87–97. New York: St. Martin's Press.

Hoopes, D. 1981. "Intercultural Communication Concepts and the Psychology of Intercultural Experience," in *Multicultural Education*. M. Pusch, ed. 10–38. New York: Intercultural Press.

Horowitz, M., J. Rosensweig, and C. Jones. 2007. "Medical Tourism: Globalization of the Healthcare Marketplace." http://www.ncbi.nlm.nih.gov (November 13; accessed January 21, 2010).

Hospital Discharge Survey. 2009. Hysterectomy Surveillance—United States, 1994–1999. CDC Report no. 7. http://www.cdc.gov/mmwr/preview/mmwrhtml/ss5105a1.htm (accessed November 18, 2009).

Hoyert, D. L., H. C. Kung, and B. L. Smith. 2005. "Deaths: Preliminary Data for 2003." *National Vital Statistics Report* Feb. 28, 53(15): 1–48.

Hufford, D. 1992. "Folk Medicine in Contemporary America," in *Herbal and Magical Medicine: Traditional Healing Today*. J. Kirkland, H. Matthews, C. W. Sullivan III, and K. Baldwin, eds. 14–31. Durham, NC: Duke University Press.

———. 1994. "Folklore and Medicine," in *Putting Folklore to Use*. M. Jones, ed. 117–35. Lexington: University Press of Kentucky.

Hutchinson, J. 1993. "Delayed Diagnosis of HIV/AIDS Among Women in the United States: Its Causes and Health Repercussions." Unpublished manuscript in files of the author.

Imershein, A., ed. 1981. *Challenges and Innovations in U.S. Health Care*. Boulder, CO: Westview Press.

Isaacs, S. L., and S. A. Schroeder. 2004. "Class—The Ignored Determinant of the Nation's Health." *New England Journal of Medicine*, 351(11): 1137–42.

Janzen, J. M. 1978. *The Quest for Therapy: Medical Pluralism in Lower Zaire*. Los Angeles: University of California Press.

Johnsen, D. 1987. "A New Threat to Pregnant Women's Autonomy." *The Hastings Center Report* 17(August/September): 33–40.

Johnson, A. 1996. *Science, Technology and Medicine. Human Arrangements: An Introduction to Sociology*, 4th ed. Dubuque, IA: Brown and Benchmark.

Johnson, M. 1987. *The Body in the Mind*. Chicago: University of Chicago Press.

Joint United Nations Programme on AIDS. 2008. *Report on the Global HIV/AIDS Epidemic 2008*. Geneva, Switzerland: Joint United Nations Programme on AIDS.

Jones, J. 1992. "The Tuskegee Legacy: AIDS and the Black Community." *Hastings Center Report* 22(6): 38–40.

Jordan, B. 1993. *Birth in Four Cultures: A Crosscultural Investigation of Childbirth in Yucatan, Holland, Sweden, and the United States*, 4th ed., revised and expanded by Robbie Davis-Floyd. Prospect Heights, IL: Waveland Press.

Journal of the American Medical Association. 1993. "Update: Acquired Immunodeficiency Syndrome—United States, 1992." 270(8): 930–31.

Julia, M., ed. 1996. *Multicultural Awareness in the Health Care Professions*. Boston: Allyn and Bacon.

Kalish, R., and D. Reynolds. 1981. *Death and Ethnicity: A Psychocultural Study*. Farmingdale, NY: Baywood.

Kam, K. (2006). "What Is Integrative Medicine? Experts Explore New Ways to Treat the Mind, Body, and Spirit—All at the Same Time." WebMD, Inc. http://www.webmd.com/cancer/integrative-med-cancer-7/integrative-care.

Kaptchuk, T. 1996. "Historical Context of the Concept of Vitalism in Complementary and Alternative Medicine," in *Fundamentals of Complementary and Alternative Medicine*. M. Micozzi, ed. 35–48. New York: Churchill Livingstone.

Kart, C. 1990. *The Realities of Aging: An Introduction to Gerontology*, 3rd ed. Boston: Allyn and Bacon.

Katchadourian, H. 1978. "Medical Perspectives on Adulthood," in *Adulthood*. E. Erikson, ed. 33–60. New York: Norton.

Kaufert, P. 1986. "Menstruation and Menstrual Change: Women in Midlife," in *Culture, Society, and Menstruation*. V. Olesen and N. F. Woods, eds. 63–76. New York: Hemisphere.

Kaufman, S. 1993. *The Healer's Tale*. Madison: University of Wisconsin Press.

Kavanagh, K., and P. Kennedy. 1992. *Promoting Cultural Diversity Strategies for Health Care Professionals*. Newbury Park, CA: Sage.

Kaw, E. 1993. Medicalization of Racial Features: Asian American Women and Cosmetic Surgery. *Medical Anthropology Quarterly* 7(1): 74–89.

Keckley, P. H., and L. L. Eselius. 2009. "2009 Survey of Health Care Consumers Key Findings, Strategic Implications." Washington, DC: Deloitte Center for Health Solutions, Deloitte Development LLC.,

Keckley, P. H., and H. R. Underwood. (2008). *Medical Tourism: Consumers in Search of Value*. Washington, DC: Deloitte Center for Health Solutions.

Kegeles, S., N. Adler, and C. Irwin. 1988. "Sexually Active Adolescents and Condoms: Changes Over One Year in Knowledge, Attitudes and Use." *American Journal of Public Health* 78: 460–67.

Keshavarz, H., S. Hillis, B. Kieke, and P. Marchbanks. 2002. "Hysterectomy Surveillance—U.S., 1994–1999. Rept. No: SS-5 (July 12, 2002). Atlanta: Centers for Disease Control.

Kessels, R. P. C. (2003). "Patients' Memory for Medical Information." *Journal of the Royal Society of Medicine* 96(5): 219–22.

Kidder, T. (2003). *Mountains Beyond Mountains: The Quest of Dr. Paul Farmer, a Man Who Would Cure the World*. New York: Random House.

Kinsey, A., W. Pomeroy, and C. Martin. 1948. *Sexual Behavior in the Human Male*. Philadelphia: Saunders.

———. 1953. *Sexual Behavior in the Human Female*. Philadelphia: Saunders.

Kinsey, K. 1994. " 'But I Know My Man': HIV/AIDS Risk Appraisals and Heuristical Reasoning Patterns among Childbearing Women." *Holistic Nurse Practitioner* 8(2): 79–88.

Kissell, J. 2009. "Justness, Health Care, and Health Disparities," in *Cultural Proficiency in Addressing Health Disparities*. S. Kosoko-Lasaki, C. Cook, and R. O'Brien, eds. 57–71. Sudbury, MA: Jones and Bartlett.

Kleinman, A. 1980. *Patients and Healers in the Context of Culture: An Exploration of the Borderland between Anthropology, Medicine, and Psychiatry*. Los Angeles: University of California Press.

Kleinman, A. (1980). *Patients and Healers in the Context of Culture: An Exploration of the Borderland between Anthropology, Medicine, and Psychiatry*. Los Angeles: University of California Press.

———. 1984. "Indigenous Systems of Healing: Questions for Professional, Popular, and Folk Care," in *Alternative Medicines: Popular and Policy Perspectives*. J. Salmon, ed. 138–64. New York: Tavistock.

———. 1986a. "Concepts and a Model for the Comparison of Medical Systems as Cultural Systems," in *Concepts of Health, Illness and Disease: A Comparative Perspective*. C. Currer and M. Stacey, eds. 29–47. Oxford: Berg.

———. 1986b. *Social Origins of Distress and Disease*. New Haven, CT: Yale University Press.

Kleinman, A., L. Eisenberg, and B. Good. (1978). "Culture, Illness, and Care: Clinical Lessons from Anthropologic and Cross-Cultural Research." *Annals of Internal Medicine* 88: 251–58.

Kleinman, J., and J. Madans. 1985. "The Effects of Maternal Smoking, Physical Stature, and Educational Attainment on the Incidence of Low Birth Weight." *American Journal of Epidemiology* 121(6): 832–55.

Korbin, J. 1987. "Child Abuse and Neglect: The Cultural Context," in *The Battered Child*, 4th ed. R. Helfer and R. Kempe, eds. 23–41. Chicago: University of Chicago Press.

Korbin, J., and M. Johnston. 1982. "Steps Toward Resolving Cultural Conflict in a Pediatric Hospital." *Clinical Pediatrics* 21(5): 259–63.

Kornblum, W., and J. Julian. 1995. *Social Problems*, 8th ed. Englewood Cliffs, NJ: Prentice-Hall.

Kosoko-Lasaki, S., C. Cook, and R. O'Brien, eds. 2009. *Cultural Proficiency in Addressing Health Disparities*. Sudbury, MA: Jones and Bartlett.

Krause, E. 1977. *Power and Illness: The Political Sociology of Health and Medical Care*. New York: Elsevier.

Kreps, G., and E. Knuimoto. 1994. *Effective Communication in Multicultural Health Settings*. Thousand Oaks, CA: Sage.

Krieger, D. 1984. "Therapeutic Touch and the Metaphysics of Nursing," in *Mind, Body and Health: Toward an Integral Medicine*. J. Gordon, D. Jaffe, and D. Bresler, eds. 107–16. New York: Human Sciences Press.

Krugman, P. (2009). "Health Care Realities." *New York Times*, July 31, national edition, sec. 1.

Kunitz, S. 1983. *Disease Change and the Role of Medicine: The Navajo Experience*. Berkeley: University of California Press.

———. 1994. *Disease and Social Diversity: The European Impact on the Health of Non-Europeans*. New York: Oxford University Press.

Kurth, A., and M. Hutchinson. 1989. "A Context for HIV Testing in Pregnancy." *Journal of Nurse-Midwifery* 34(5): 259–65.

LaFleur, W. 1992. *Liquid Life: Abortion and Buddhism in Japan*. Princeton, NJ: Princeton University Press.

Laguerre, M. 1987. *Afro-Caribbean Folk Medicine*. South Hadley, MA: Bergin and Garvey.

Laine, C., and F. Davidoff. 1996. "Patient-centered Medicine: A Professional Evolution." *Journal of the American Medical Association* 275(2): 152–56.

Lakan, S., E. Hamlat, T. McNamee, and C. Laird. 2009. "Time for a Unified Approach to Medical Ethics." *Philosophy, Ethics, and Humanities in Medicine* 4(13): 1–6. http://www.peh-med.com/content/4/1/13 (accessed January 14, 2010)

Lakoff, G. 1987. *Women, Fire, and Dangerous Things*. Chicago: University of Chicago Press.

Lambert, H. (2006). "Accounting for EBM: Notions of Evidence in Medicine." *Social Science & Medicine* 62(11): 2633–45.

Lambert, H., E. J. Gordon, and E. A. Bogdan-Lovis,. (2006). "Introduction: Gift Horse or Trojan Horse? Social Science Perspectives on Evidence-based Health Care." *Social Science & Medicine* 62(11): 2613–20.

Landy, D., ed. 1977. *Culture, Disease, and Healing: Studies in Medical Anthropology*. New York: Macmillan.

Laqueur, T. 1990. *Making Sex: Body and Gender from the Greeks to Freud*. Cambridge, MA: Harvard University Press.

Leichliter, J. S., A. Chandra, N. Liddon, K. A. Fenton, and S. O. Aral. 2007. "Prevalence and Correlates of Heterosexual Anal and Oral Sex in Adolescents and Adults in the United States." *Journal of Infectious Diseases* 196: 1852–59.

Leininger, M. 1985. "Transcultural Caring: A Different Way to Help People," in *Handbook of Cross-Cultural Counseling and Therapy*. P. Pedersen, ed. 107–16. Westport, CT: Greenwood.

———. 1993. "Assumptive Premises of the Theory," in *Cultural Care Diversity and Universality Theory*. M. Leininger and C. Reynolds, eds. 15–30. Newbury Park, CA: Sage.

———. 2002. "Culture Care Theory: A Major Contribution to Advance Transcultural Nursing Knowledge and Practices." *Journal of Transcultural Nursing* 13(3): 189–92.

Lempert, David. 2007. "Women's Increasing Wage Penalties from Being Overweight and Obese." Bureau of Labor Statistics Working Paper no. 414, December.

Leslie, C. 1976. "Introduction," in *Asian Medical Systems: A Comparative Study*. C. Leslie, ed. 1–12. Los Angeles: University of California Press.

Lester, C., and L. Saxxon. 1988. "AIDS in the Black Community: The Plague, the Politics, the People." *Death Studies* 12: 563–71.

Lewis, D., and J. Watters. 1989. "Human Immunodeficiency Virus Seroprevalence in Female Intravenous Drug Users: The Puzzle of Black Women's Risk." *Social Science and Medicine* 29(9): 1071–76.

Lewis, G. 1986. "Concepts of Health and Illness in a Sepik Society," in *Concepts of Health, Illness and Disease: A Comparative Perspective*. C. Currer and M. Stacey, eds. 119–35. Oxford: Berg.

Lieberman, J. 1970. *The Tyranny of the Experts: How Professionals Are Closing the Open Society*. New York: Walker.

Liebow, E. 1967. *Tally's Corner: A Study of Negro Streetcorner Men*. Boston: Little, Brown.

Like, R. C. 2005. "Culturally Competent Family Medicine: Transforming Clinical Practice and Ourselves." *American Family Physician* 72(11): 2189–99.

Limandri, B. 1989. "Disclosure of Stigmatizing Conditions: The Discloser's Perspective." *Archives of Psychiatric Nursing* 3(2): 69–78.

Lipman, T. (2000). "Power and Influence in Clinical Effectiveness and Evidence-based Medicine." *Family Practice* 17(6): 557–63.

Lippman, A. 1991. "Prenatal Genetic Testing and Screening: Constructing Needs and Reinforcing Inequities." *American Journal of Law and Medicine* 17: 17.

Lock, M. 1988. "Introduction," in *Biomedicine Examined*. M. Lock and D. Gordon, eds. 3–16. Dordrecht, Netherlands: Academic.

———. 1993. "The Politics of Mid-Life and Menopause," in *Knowledge, Power, and Practice: The Anthropology of Medicine and Everyday Life*. S. Lindenbaum and M. Lock, eds. 330–63. Berkeley: University of California Press.

———. (2002). *Twice Dead: Organ Transplants and the Reinvention of Death*. Los Angeles: University of California Press.

Locke, D. 1992. *Increasing Multicultural Understanding: A Comprehensive Model*. Newbury Park, CA: Sage.

Logan, M. 1977. "Humoral Medicine in Guatemala and Peasant Acceptance of Modern Medicine," in *Culture, Disease, and Healing: Studies in Medical Anthropology*. D. Landy, ed. 487–95. New York: Macmillan.

Loustaunau, M. 1990. "Folk Medicine in the Mesilla Valley." *The World and I* 5(2): 654–65.

Lowenberg, J. 1989. *Caring and Responsibility*. Philadelphia: University of Pennsylvania Press.

Luecke, R. 1993. "A New Dawn with Fingers to the World," in *A New Dawn in Guatemala: Toward a Worldwide Health Vision*. R. Luecke, ed. ix–xx. Prospect Heights, IL: Waveland Press.

Lupton, D. 1994. *Medicine as Culture: Illness, Disease and the Body in Western Societies*. London: Sage.

Lyng, S. 1990. *Holistic Health and Biomedical Medicine*. Albany: State University of New York Press.

MacDorman, M., and T. Mathews. (2008). *Recent Trends in Infant Mortality in the United States*. NCHS data brief, no 9. Hyattsville, MD: National Center for Health Statistics.

Macintyre, S., and D. Oldman. 1977. "Coping with Migraine," in *Medical Encounters: The Experience of Illness and Treatment*. A. Davis and G. Horobin, eds. 55–71. New York: St. Martin's Press.

Mack, T., and R. Ross. 1989. "Risks and Benefits of Long-Term Treatment with Estrogens." *Schweizensche Medizinische Wochenschrift* 119: 1811–20.

Magner, L. 1992. *A History of Medicine*. New York: Marcel Dekker.

Magrane, D., and J. Lang. 2006. "An Overview of Women in U.S. Academic Medicine, 2005–06. Analysis In Brief (October) 6(7). http://www.aamc.org/data/aib/aibissues/aibvol6_no7.pdf.

Majumdar, B. 1995. *Culture and Health: Culture-Sensitive Training Manual for the Health Care Provider*, 4th ed. Hamilton, Ontario: McMaster University.

Manio, E., and R. Hall. 1987. "Asian Family Traditions and Their Influence in Transcultural Health Care Delivery." *Children's Health Care* 15: 172–77.

Marmot, M. 2002. "The Influence of Income on Health: Views of an Epidemiologist." *Health Affairs* 21(2): 31–46.

Marmot, M., M. Shipley, and G. Rose. 1984. "Inequalities in Death—Specific Explanations of a General Pattern." *Lancet* 83: 1003–1006.

Martin, E. 1987. *The Woman in the Body: A Cultural Analysis of Reproduction*. Boston: Beacon Press.

———. 1990. "Toward an Anthropology of Immunology: The Body as Nation State." *Medical Anthropology Quarterly* 4(4): 410–26.

———. 1994. *Flexible Bodies: Tracking Immunity in American Culture from the Days of Polio to the Age of AIDS*. Boston: Beacon Press.

Martínez-Donate, A. P., J. A. Zellner, J. A. Fernández-Cerdeño, F. Sañudo, F. Melbourne, F. Hovell, C. L. Sipan, M. Engelberg, and M. Ji. (2009). "Hombres Sanos: Exposure and Response to a Social Marketing HIV Prevention Campaign Targeting Heterosexually Identified Latino Men Who Have Sex with Men and Women." *AIDS Education and Prevention* 21(Suppl. B): 124–36.

Masters, W., and V. Johnson. 1966. *Human Sexual Response*. Boston: Little, Brown.

Maternowska, C. (2009). "Truck Stop Girls," *New York Times Sunday Magazine*, August 23.

Mays, V., and S. Cochran. 1987. "Acquired Immunodeficiency Syndrome and Black Americans: Special Psychosocial Issues." *Public Health Reports* 102(2): 224–31.

Mays, V., S. Cochran, and N. Barnes. (2007). "Race, Race-based Discrimination, and Health Outcomes among African Americans." *Annual Review of Psychology* 58: 201–25.

McCormick, R. 1994. "Beyond Principalism Is Not Enough," in *A Matter of Principles?: Ferment in U.S. Bioethics*. E. DuBose, R. Hamel, and L. O'Connell, eds. 344–61. Valley Forge, PA: Trinity Press International.

McKenna, J. J., and T. McDade. (2005). "Why Babies Should Never Sleep Alone: A Review of the Co-Sleeping Controversy in Relation to SIDS, Bedsharing and Breast feeding." *Paediatric Respiratory Reviews* 6: 134–52.

McKnight, J. 1993. "Taking Charge of Health in a Chicago Neighborhood," in *A New Dawn in Guatemala: Toward a Worldwide Health Vision*. R. Luecke, ed. 219–27. Prospect Heights, IL: Waveland Press.

McLean, A. 2007. *The Person in Dementia: A Study of Nursing Home Care in the US*. Toronto: Broadview Press

McQuillan, G., M. Khare, T. Ezzati-Rice, J. Karon, C. Schable, and R. Murphy. 1994. "The Seroepidemiology of Human Immunodeficiency Virus in the United States Household Population: NHANES III, 1988–1991." *Journal of Acquired Immune Deficiency Syndrome* 7(11): 1195–1201.

Mead, M. 1963 [1928]. *Coming of Age in Samoa: A Study of Adolescence and Sex in Primitive Society*. New York: Mentor Books.

Mechanic, D. 1962. "The Concept of Illness Behavior." *Journal of Chronic Diseases* 15: 189–94.

———. 1978. *Medical Sociology*, 2nd ed. New York: Free Press.

———. 2004. "The Rise and Fall of Managed Care." *Journal of Health and Social Behavior* 45(Suppl.): 76–86.

———. 2006. *The Truth about Health Care: Why Reform Is Not Working in America.* New Brunswick, NJ: Rutgers University Press.

Meigs, A. 1983. *Food, Sex, and Pollution: A New Guinea Religion.* New Brunswick, NJ: Rutgers University Press.

Messina, S. 1992. *Lesbian, Gay and Bisexual Youth: At Risk and Underserved.* Washington, DC: Center for Population Options.

Micozzi, M. 1996a. "Characteristics of Complementary and Alternative Medicine Systems," in *Fundamentals of Complementary and Alternative Medicine.* M. Micozzi, ed. 3–8. New York: Churchill Livingstone.

———. 1996b. *Fundamentals of Complementary and Alternative Medicine.* New York: Churchill Livingstone.

Milstein, A., and M. Smith. (2006). America's New Refugees—Seeking Affordable Surgery Offshore. *New England Journal of Medicine* 355(16): 1637–40.

Moerman, D. 2002. *Meaning, Medicine, and the "Placebo Effect."* Cambridge: University of Cambridge Press.

Money, J. 1981. *Love and Love Sickness: The Science of Sex, Gender Difference, and Pair-Bonding.* Baltimore: Johns Hopkins University Press.

Montagu, A. 1969. "Letters to the Editor." *New York Times* (July 13): E-13.

Monthly Forum on Women in Higher Education. 1995. 1(3): 6–7.

Moore, L., P. van Arsdale, J. Glittenberg, and R. Aldrich. 1980. *The Biocultural Basis of Health: Expanding Views of Medical Anthropology.* Prospect Heights, IL: Waveland Press.

Morgan, L. 1989. "When Does Life Begin? A Cross-Cultural Perspective on the Personhood of Fetuses and Young Children," in *Abortion Rights and Fetal "Personhood."* E. Doerr and J. Prescott, eds. 97–114. Long Beach, CA: Centerline Press.

Morgan, M. M., J. Goodson, and G. O. Barnett. (1998). "Long-Term Changes in Compliance with Clinical Guidelines through Computer-based Reminders," in *Proceedings of the AMIA Symposium.* 493–97. Bethesda, MD: AMIA Symposium, American Medical Informatics Association.

Morley, P. 1978. "Culture and the Cognitive World of Traditional Medical Beliefs: Some Preliminary Considerations," in *Culture and Curing: Anthropological Perspectives on Traditional Medical Beliefs and Practices.* P. Morley and R. Wallis, eds. 1–18. Pittsburgh: University of Pittsburgh Press.

Morrissey, S., ed. 2008. "Health of the Nation—Coverage for All Americans." *New England Journal of Medicine* 359(8): 777–80.

Muller, J., and B. Koenig. 1988. "On the Boundary of Life and Death: The Definition of Dying by Medical Residents," in *Biomedicine Examined.* M. Lock and D. Gordon, eds. 351–74. Dordrecht, Netherlands: Kluwer Academic.

Mumford, E. 1983. *Medical Sociology: Patients, Providers, and Policies.* New York: Random House.

Munson, R. 2000. *Intervention and Reflection*, 6th ed. Belmont, CA: Wadsworth.

Myrdal, G. 1944. *An American Dilemma: The Negro Problem and Modern Democracy.* New York: Harper.

Nachtigall, L. 1990. "Hormone Replacement Therapy," in *Highlights from the Sixth International Congress on the Menopause*. CT: Beardsley and Co.

Naisbitt, J., and P. Aburdene. 1990. *Megatrends 2000: Ten New Directions for the 1990's*. New York: Morrow.

National Center for Complementary and Alternative Medicine. 2008. *The Use of Complementary and Alternative Medicine in the United States*. Washington, DC: National Institutes of Health.

National Poverty Center. 2006. "Poverty Facts: Poverty in the United States— Frequently Asked Questions." University of Michigan, Gerald R. Ford School of Public Policy. http://www.npc.umich.edu/poverty.

National Women's Health Network. 2007. "Feminine Forever Becomes Young at Heart." http://www.nwhn.org/alerts/details (accessed November 17, 2009).

———. 2008. "Natural Hormones at Menopause." http://www.nwhn.org/healthinfo/details (accessed November 17, 2009).

National Center for Health Statistics. 1988. *Health, United States, 1987*. Washington, DC: U.S. Government Printing Office.

———. 1991. *Disability and Health: Characteristics of Persons by Limitation of Activity and Assessed Health Status, United States, 1984–88*. Advance Data, no. 197. Washington, DC: U.S. Government Printing Office.

———. 2009. Table 98. "Prescription Drug Use in the Past Month By Sex, Age, Race and Hispanic Origin: United States, 1988–1994 and 2001–2004." *Health, United States, 2008, with Chartbook*. Hyattsville MD: U.S. Department of Health and Human Services.

Navarro, V. 1977. *Medicine Under Capitalism*. New York: Prodist.

———. 1994. "Race or Class versus Race and Class: Mortality Differentials in the United States," in *Issues in Medical Sociology*, 3rd ed. H. Schwartz, ed. 491–504. New York: McGraw-Hill.

Newport, F. (2007). "Average American Weighs 17 Pounds More Than 'Ideal.' " *Gallup Daily News: Well-Being*. Gallup, Inc. http://www.gallup.com/poll/wellbeing.aspx.

Ngalande, R. C., J. Levy, C. P. N. Kapondo, and R. C. Bailey. (2006). "Acceptability of Male Circumcision for Prevention of HIV Infection in Malawi." *AIDS and Behavior* 10(4): 377–85.

Nichols, M. 1990. "Women and Acquired Immunodeficiency Syndrome: Issues for Prevention," in *AIDS and Sex: An Integrated Biomedical and Biobehavioral Approach*. B. Voeller, J. Reinisch, and M. Gottlieb, eds. 375–92. New York: Oxford University Press.

Nisbett, R. E. 2005. "Heredity, Environment, and Race Differences in IQ: A Commentary on Rushton and Jensen." *Psychology, Public Policy, and Law* 11(2): 302–10.

Norris, A. 2002. *Essentials of Telemedicine and Telecare*. Chichester, UK: Wiley.

Novak, D., G. Volk, D. Drossman, and M. Lipkin. 1993. "Medical Interviewing and Interpersonal Skills Teaching in U.S. Medical Schools." *Journal of the American Medical Association* 269: 2102–5.

Nunley, M. 1995. "The Bell Curve: Too Smooth to Be True." *American Behavioral Scientist* 39(1): 74–83.

Nyamathi, A., P. Shuler, and M. Porche. 1990. "AIDS Educational Program for Minority Women at Risk." *Family and Community Health* 13(2): 54–64.

O'Connor, B. B. 1995. *Healing Traditions: Alternative Medicine and the Health Professions*. Philadelphia: University of Pennsylvania Press.

Office of Minority Health. 2005. *What Is Cultural Competency?* Rockville, MD: Health Resources and Services Administration.

Office of Minority Health & Health Disparities. 2007. *Eliminate Disparities in Infant Mortality.* Atlanta: Centers for Disease Control and Prevention.

Ogburn, W. 1937. *Social Change with Respect to Culture and Original Nature.* New York: Viking Press.

Oliver, W. 1989. "Sexual Conquest and Patterns of Black-on-Black Violence: A Structural-Cultural Perspective." *Violence and Victims* 4(4): 257–73.

Omer, S. B., D. A. Salmon, W. A. Orenstein, M. P. Dehart, and N. Halsey. (2009). "Vaccine Refusal, Mandatory Immunization, and the Risks of Vaccine-Preventable Diseases." *New England Journal of Medicine* 360(19): 1981.

Pachter, L. 1994. "Folk Illness Beliefs and Behaviors and Their Implication for Health Care Delivery." *Journal of the American Medical Association* 271(9): 690.

Pamies, R., and P. Nsiah-Kumi. 2009. "Addressing Health Disparities in the 21st Century," in *Cultural Proficiency in Addressing Health Disparities.* S. Kosoko-Lasaki, C. Cook, and R. O'Brien, eds. 1–23. Sudbury, MA: Jones and Bartlett.

Pappas, G., et al. 1993. "The Increasing Disparity in Mortality Between Socioeconomic Groups in the United States, 1960 and 1986." *New England Journal of Medicine* 329(July 8): 103–09.

Parsons, T. 1951. *The Social System.* Glencoe, IL: Free Press.

Partners in Health. 2009. "The PIH Vision: Whatever It Takes." http://www.pih.org/who/vision.html.

Payer, L. 1988. *Medicine and Culture.* New York: Penguin Books.

———. 1996. *Medicine and Culture: Varieties of Treatments in the United States, England, West Germany and France.* New York: Henry Holt.

Pelto, P., and G. Pelto. 1996. "Field Methods in Medical Anthropology," in *Medical Anthropology: Contemporary Theory and Method.* T. Johnson and C. Sargent, eds. 293–324. New York: Praeger.

Perez, M., and R. Luquis, eds. 2008. *Cultural Competence in Health Education and Health Promotion.* San Francisco: Jossey-Bass.

Pescosolido, B., and C. Boyer. 2005. "The American Health Care System: Entering the Twenty-first Century with High Risk, Major Challenges, and Great Opportunities," in *The Blackwell Companion to Medical Sociology.* W. Cockerham, ed. 177–98. Oxford: Blackwell.

Pfifferling, J. 1981. "A Cultural Prescription for Medicocentrism," in *The Relevance of Social Science for Medicine.* L. Eisenberg and A. Kleinman, eds. 197–222. Dordrecht, Netherlands: D. Reidel.

Philipsen, G. 2003. "Cultural Communication," in *Cross-Cultural and Intercultural Communication,* 2nd ed. W. Gudykunst, ed. 35–51. Thousand Oaks, CA: Sage.

Pickin, C., and S. St. Leger. 1993. *Assessing Health Need Using the Life Cycle Framework.* Buckingham, UK: Open University Press.

Pierret, J. 1995 [1983]. "The Social Meanings of Health: Paris, the Essone and the Herault," in *The Meaning of Illness: Anthropology, History and Sociology.* M. Augé and C. Herzlich, eds. 151–73. Translated from the French by K. Durnin, C. Lambein, K. Leclercq-Jones, B. Garnier, and R. Williams. London: Harwood Academic Publishers.

Pivnick, A. 1993. "HIV Infection and the Meaning of Condoms." *Culture, Medicine, and Psychiatry* 17(4): 431–53.

Polednak, A. 1989. *Racial and Ethnic Differences in Disease*. New York: Oxford University Press.

Potts, M., D. T. Halperin, D. Kirby, A. Swidler, E. Marseille, J. D. Klausner, N. Hearst, R. G. Wamai, J. G. Kahn, and J. Walsh. (2008). "Reassessing HIV Prevention." *Science* 320(5877): 749–50.

Pratt, L. 1976. *Family Structure and Effective Health Behavior: The Energized Family*. Boston: Houghton Mifflin.

Prohaska, T., G. Albrecht, and J. Levy. 1990. "Determinants of Self-Perceived Risk for AIDS." *Journal of Health and Social Behavior* 31: 384–94.

Prussing, E., E. J. Sobo, E. Walker, K. Dennis, P. S. Kurtin. (2004). Communicating about Complementary/Alternative Medicine: Perspectives from Parents of Children with Down Syndrome. *Ambulatory Pediatrics* 4(6): 488–94.

———. (2005). "Between 'Desperation' and Disability Rights: A Narrative Analysis of Complementary/Alternative Medicine Use by Parents for Children with Down Syndrome." *Social Science and Medicine* 60(3): 587–98.

Public Health Service, U.S. Department of Health and Human Services. 1992. *Healthy People 2000: National Health Promotion and Disease Prevention Objectives*. Boston: Jones and Bartlett.

Quimby, E. 1992. "Anthropological Witnessing for African-Americans: Power, Responsibility, and Choice in the Age of AIDS," in *The Time of AIDS: Social Analysis, Theory, and Method*. G. Herdt and S. Lindenbaum, eds. 159–84. Newbury Park, CA: Sage.

Ratliff, S. 1996. "The Multicultural Challenge to Health Care," in *Multicultural Awareness in the Health Professions*. M. Julia, ed. 162–76. Boston: Allyn and Bacon.

Reid, I. 1989. *Social Class Differences in Britain*, 3rd ed. Glasgow: Fontana Press.

Rensberger, B. 1993. "Teenage Girls Are on the 'Leading Edge' of the AIDS Scourge." *Washington Post National Weekly Edition*, August 9–15, 34.

Rice, D. 1990. "The Medical Care System: Past Trends and Future Projections," in *The Nation's Health*, 3rd ed. P. Lee and C. Estes, eds. 72–93. Boston: Jones and Bartlett.

Richardson, L. 1988. *The Dynamics of Sex and Gender: A Sociological Perspective*. New York: Harper and Row.

Rieker, P., and C. Bird. 2000. "Sociological Explanations of Gender Differences in Mental and Physical Health," in *Handbook of Medical Sociology*, 5th ed. C. Bird and A. Fremont, eds. 98–113. Upper Saddle River, NJ: Prentice Hall.

Ring, J., J. Nyquist, S. Mitchell, H. Flores, and L. Samaniego, eds. 2008. *Curriculum for Culturally Responsive Health Care: The Step-by-Step Guide for Cultural Competence Training*. New York: Radcliffe.

Rivera, G., Jr. 1990. "AIDS and Mexican Folk Medicine." *Sociology and Social Research* 75(1): 3–7.

Robertson, L., and M. Heagarty. 1975. *Medical Sociology: A General Systems Approach*. Chicago: Nelson-Hall.

Romalis, S., ed. 1981. *Childbirth: Alternatives to Medical Control*. Austin: University of Texas Press.

Romanucci-Ross, L. 1977 [1969]. "The Hierarchy of Resort in Curative Practices: The Admiralty Islands, Melanesia," in *Culture, Disease, and Healing: Studies in Medical Anthropology*. D. Landy, ed. 481–87. New York: Macmillan.

Roscoe, W. (1992). *The Zuni Man-Woman*. Albuquerque: University of New Mexico Press.

Rose, S. M., and S. Hatzenbuehler. (2009). Embodying Social Class—The Link between Poverty, Income Inequality and Health. *International Social Work* 52(4): 459–71.

Rosen, G. 1974. *From Medical Police to Social Medicine: Essays on the History of Health Care*. New York: Science History Publications.

Rosenberg, C. 2007. *Our Present Complaint: American Medicine, Then and Now*. Baltimore: Johns Hopkins University Press.

Rosenstock, I. 1966. "Why People Use Health Services." *Milbank Memorial Fund Quarterly* 44: 94–127.

Rothman, B. 1994. "Midwives in Transition: The Structure of a Clinical Revolution," in *Dominant Issues in Medical Sociology*, 3rd ed. H. Schwartz, ed. 104–12. New York: McGraw-Hill.

Russo, C., L. W. Allison, and C. Steiner. 2009. "Statistical Brief #71: Hospitalizations Related to Childbirth, 2006," in *Healthcare Cost and Utilization Project*. Agency for Healthcare Research and Quality, Rockville, MD.

Sackett, D. L., W. M. C. Rosenberg, J. A. M. Gray, R. B. Haynes, and W. S. Richardson. (1996). "Evidence Based Medicine: What It Is and What It Isn't. *British Medical Journal* 312: 71–72.

Sacks, K. 1974. "Engels Revisited: Women, the Organization of Production, and Private Property," in *Women, Culture, and Society*. M. Rosaldo and L. Lamphere, eds. 207–22. Stanford, CA: Stanford University Press.

Salmon, J., ed. 1984. *Alternative Medicines: Popular and Policy Perspectives*. New York: Routledge.

Sanders, G. D., A. M. Bayoumi, V. Sundaram, S. P. Bilir, C. P. Neukermans, C. E. Rydzak, L. R. Douglass, L. C. Lazzeroni, M. Holodniy, and D. K. Owens. (2005). "Cost-Effectiveness of Screening for HIV in the Era of Highly Active Antiretroviral Therapy." *New England Journal of Medicine* 352(6): 570–85.

Sargent, C., and N. Stark. (1989). "Childbirth Education and Childbirth Models: Parental Perspectives on Control, Anesthesia, and Technological Intervention in the Birth Process." *Medical Anthropology Quarterly* 3(1): 36–51.

Schaefer, R. 2000. *Sociology: A Brief Introduction*, 3rd ed.. New York: McGraw-Hill.

Schlegel, A., and H. Barry III. 1991. *Adolescence: An Anthropological Inquiry*. New York: Free Press.

Schlesinger, A., Jr. 1992. *The Disuniting of America*. New York: Norton.

Schmidt, D. 1978. "The Family as the Unit of Medical Care." *Journal of Family Practice* 7(2): 303–13.

Schoenborn, C., S. Marsh, and A. Hardy. 1994. "AIDS Knowledge and Attitudes for 1992: Data from the National Health Interview Survey," in *Advance Data from Vital and Health Statistics, No. 243*. Hyattsville, MD: National Center for Health Statistics.

Schweitzer, M. 1983. "The Elders: Cultural Dimensions of Aging in Two American Indian Communities," in *Growing Old in Different Societies*. J. Sokolovsky, ed. 168–78. Belmont, CA: Wadsworth.

Scully, D., and P. Bart. 1979. "A Funny Thing Happened on the Way to the Orifice: Women in Gynecology Textbooks," in *The Cultural Crisis of Modern Medicine*. J. Ehrenreich, ed. 212–26. New York: Monthly Review Press.

Sharp, L. (2006). *Strange Harvest: Organ Transplants, Denatured Bodies, and the Transformed Self*. Los Angeles: University of California Press.

Shorter, E. 1985. *Bedside Manners*. New York: Simon and Schuster.

Shryock, R. 1966. "The American Physician in 1846 and in 1946: A Study in Professional Contrasts," in *Medicine in America: Historical Essays*. R. Shryock, ed. 149–76. Baltimore: Johns Hopkins University Press.

Shweder, R. 1991. *Thinking Through Cultures: Expeditions in Cultural Psychology*. Cambridge, MA: Harvard University Press.

Sigerist, H. 1960 [1947]. "Medical History in the United States: Past-Future," in *On the History of Medicine*. F. Marti-Ibanez, ed. 233–50. New York: MD Publications.

Silenzio, V. M., J. B. Pena, P. R. Duberstein, J. Cerel, and K. L. Knox. (2007). "Sexual Orientation and Risk Factors for Suicidal Ideation and Suicide Attempts among Adolescents and Young Adults." *American Journal of Public Health* 97(11): 2017–19.

Singer, M. 1995. "Beyond the Ivory Tower: Critical Praxis in Medical Anthropology." *Medical Anthropology Quarterly* 9(1): 80–106.

———. (2009). *Introduction to Syndemics: A Critical Systems Approach to Public and Community Health*. San Francisco: Jossey Bass.

Singer, M., F. Valentin, H. Baer, and Z. Jia. 1992. "Why Does Juan Garcia Have a Drinking Problem? The Perspective of Critical Medical Anthropology." *Medical Anthropology* 14(1): 77–108.

Slataper, R. 1997. "Quality of Care and the Hospitalist." *The Hospitalist Newsletter of the National Association of Inpatient Physicians* 1: 5–6.

Slater, V. 1996. "Healing Touch," in *Fundamentals of Complementary and Alternative Medicine*. M. Micozzi, ed. 121–36. New York: Churchill Livingstone.

Smelser, N. J., W. J. Wilson, and F. Mitchell. (2001). *America Becoming: Racial Trends and Their Consequences: Volume 1*. Washington, DC: National Academy Press.

Smith, G. L. (2001). *An Ethnographic Study of Home Remedy Use for African-American Children*. Houston: University of Texas Health Science Center at Houston School of Nursing.

Smith, S., and J. M. Smith. 2010. "Rising to Meet an Infinite Need: Partners in Health, Long a Force in Haiti, Vaults into Central Role. *Boston Globe*, January 24. http://www.boston.com/bostonglobe/.

Snow, L. 1993. *Walkin' over Medicine*. Boulder, CO: Westview Press.

Snyder, A., D. McLaughlin, and J. Findeis. 2006. "Household Composition and Poverty among Female-Headed Households with Children: Differences by Race and Residence." *Rural Sociology* 71(4): 597–624.

Sobo, E. 1993. *One Blood: The Jamaican Body*. Albany: State University of New York Press.

———. 1995. *Choosing Unsafe Sex: AIDS-Risk Denial among Disadvantaged Women*. Philadelphia: University of Pennsylvania Press.

———. 1996a. "Abortion Traditions in Rural Jamaica." *Social Science and Medicine* 42(4): 495–508.

———. 1996b. The Jamaican Body's Role in Emotional Experience and Sense Perception." *Culture, Medicine and Psychiatry* 20: 313–42.

———. 1997 (1994). "The Sweetness of Fat: Health, Procreation, and Sociability in Rural Jamaica," in *Food and Culture: A Reader*. C. Counihan and P. Van Esterik, eds. New Brunswick, NJ: Rutgers University Press.

———. 1997. "Self-Disclosure and Self-Construction among HIV-Positive People: The Rhetorical Uses of Stereotypes and Sex." *Anthropology and Medicine* 4: 67–87.

———. 2003. "Prevention and Healing in the Household," in *Child Health Services Research: Applications, Innovations, and Insights*. E. J. Sobo and P. S. Kurtin, eds. 67–119. San Francisco: Jossey-Bass.

———. 2004a. "Good Communication in Pediatric Cancer Care: A Culturally-Informed Research Agenda." *Journal of Pediatric Oncology Nursing* 21(3): 150–54.

———. 2004b. "Nurses' Knowledge of Parent or Patient Communication Needs in a Pediatric Cancer Unit: Room for Improvement." *Journal of Nursing Care Quality* 19(3): 253–62.

Sobo, E. (2009a). *Culture and Meaning in Health Services Research: A Practical Field Guide*. Walnut Creek, CA: Left Coast Press.

———. 2009b. Medical Travel: What It Means and Why It Matters. *Medical Anthropology* 28(4): 326–35

Sobo, E. J. 2010. "Caring for Children with Special Healthcare Needs: 'Once We Got There, It Was Fine,'" in *Chronic Conditions, Fluid States: Globalization and the Anthropology of Illness*. L. Manderson and C. Smith-Morris, eds. 212–29. New Brunswick, NJ: Rutgers University Press.

———. In Press. "Medical Anthropology in Disciplinary Context: Definitional Struggles and Key Debates (Or: Answering the 'Cri Du Coeur')," in *A Companion to Medical Anthropology*. M. Singer and P. I. Erickson, eds. Hoboken, NJ: Blackwell.

Sobo, E. J., C. Bowman, J. Halloran, S. M. Asch, M. B. Goetz, and A. L. Gifford. (2008). " 'A Routine Thing': Clinician Strategies for Implementing HIV Testing for At-Risk Patients in a Busy Healthcare Organization (and Implications for Implementation of other New Practice Recommendations)." *Anthropology & Medicine* 15(3): 213–25.

Sobo, E. J., and M. Seid. (2003). "Cultural Issues in Health Services Delivery: What Kind of 'Competence' Is Needed, and from Whom?" *Annals of Behavioral Science & Medical Education* 9(2): 97–100.

Sobo, E. J., M. Seid, L. R. Gelhard. (2006). "Parent-identified Barriers to Pediatric Health Care: A Process-oriented Model and Method." *Health Services Research* 41(1): 148–72.

Sokol, E. 1992. "A Formula for Disaster." *Multinational Monitor* (March): 9–13.

Soroka, M., and G. Bryjak. 1995. *Social Problems: A World at Risk*. Boston: Allyn and Bacon.

Spector, R. 2000. *Cultural Diversity in Health and Illness*, 5th ed. Upper Saddle River, NJ: Prentice Hall Health.

Srivastava, R., ed. 2007. *The Healthcare Professional's Guide to Clinical Cultural Competence*. Toronto: Mosby Elsevier.

Stack, C. 1974. *All Our Kin: Strategies for Survival in a Black Community*. New York: Harper and Row.

Stanford, D. 1977. "All About Sex . . . After Middle Age." *American Journal of Nursing* 77(4): 608–11.

Stafford, A. 1978. "The Application of Clinical Anthropology to Medical Practice: Case Study of Recurrent Abdominal Pain in a Preadolescent Mexican-American Female," in *The Anthropology of Health*. E. Bauwens, ed. 12–22. St. Louis: C.V. Mosby.

Starr, P. 1982. *The Social Transformation of American Medicine*. New York: Basic Books.

Stetler, C. B., M. W. Legro, C. M. Wallace, C. Bowman, M. Guihan, H. Hagedorn, B. Kimmel, N. D. Sharp, J. L. Smith. 2006. "The Role of Formative Evaluation in Implementation Research and the QUERI Experience." *Journal of General Internal Medicine* 21(S2): S1–8.

Stine, G. 1993. *Acquired Immune Deficiency Syndrome: Biological, Medical, Social, and Legal Issues*. Englewood Cliffs, NJ: Prentice Hall.

Suchman, E. 1965. "Social Patterns of Illness and Medical Care." *Journal of Health and Human Behavior* 6: 2–16.

Sullivan, R. 1994. "Sanguine Practices: A Historical and Historiographic Reconsideration of Heroic Therapy in the Age of Rush." *Bulletin of the History of Medicine* 68: 211–34.

Syme, S., and L. Berkman. 1994. "Social Class, Susceptibility, and Sickness," in *The Sociology of Health and Illness: Critical Perspectives*, 4th ed. P. Conrad and R. Kern, eds. 29–35. New York: St. Martin's Press.

Szasz, T., and M. Hollender. 1956. "A Contribution to the Philosophy of Medicine: The Basic Models of the Doctor-Patient Relationship." *Journal of the American Medical Association* 97: 585–88.

Tanner, W., and R. Pollack. 1988. "The Effect of Condom Use and Erotic Instructions on Attitudes Toward Condoms." *Journal of Sex Research* 25(4): 537–41.

Taylor, C., and D. Lourea. 1992. "HIV Prevention: A Dramaturgical Analysis and Practical Guide to Creating Safer Sex Interventions," in *Rethinking AIDS Prevention*. R. Bolton and M. Singer, eds. 105–46. New York: Gordon and Breach Science.

Tervalon, M., and J. Murray-Garcia. 1998. "Cultural Humility versus Cultural Competence: A Critical Distinction in Defining Physician Training Outcomes in Multicultural Education." *Journal of Health Care for the Poor and Underserved* 9(2): 117–25.

Thompson, J., T. Yager, and J. Martin. 1993. "Estimated Condom Failure and Frequency of Condom Use among Gay Men." *American Journal of Public Health* 83(10): 1409–12.

Thorson, J. 2000. *Aging in a Changing Society*, 2nd ed. Philadelphia: Brunner/Mazel.

Toubia, N. 1994. "Female Circumcision as a Public Health Issue." *New England Journal of Medicine* 331(11): 712–16.

Tseng, W. S., and J. Strelzer. 2008. *Cultural Competence in Health Care*. New York: Springer.

Turner, B. 1984. *The Body and Society*. Oxford: Blackwell.

———. 1995. *Medical Power and Social Knowledge*, 2nd ed. London: Sage.

Twaddle, A. 1969. "Health Decisions and Sick Role Variations: An Exploration." *Journal of Health and Social Behavior* 10: 105–14.

Twaddle, A., and R. Hessler. 1987. *A Sociology of Health*, 2nd ed. New York: Macmillan.

Ulrich, R. S. 1984. "View through a Window May Influence Recovery from Surgery." *Science* 224(4647): 420–21.

———. 2006. Evidence-based Healthcare Architecture. *Lancet* 368(Suppl. 1): S38–39.

United Nations. 1978. *International Bill of Human Rights*. New York: United Nations.

U.S. Census Bureau. 1986. "Household Wealth and Asset Ownership: 1984." *Current Population Reports*, ser. P-70, no. 7. Washington, DC: U.S. Government Printing Office.

———. 1990. "Household and Family Characteristics: March 1990 and 1989." *Current Population Reports*, ser. P-20, no.447. Washington, DC: U.S. Government Printing Office.

———. 1993. Washington, DC: U.S. Government Printing Office.

———. 1995. Washington, DC: U.S. Government Printing Office.

———. 2007. *Statistical Abstract of the United States, 2006*. Washington, DC: U.S. Government Printing Office.

———. 2009. *2006–2008 American Community Survey 3-Year Estimates: Data Profile Highlights*. Washington, DC: U.S. Government Printing Office.

U.S. Department of Health and Human Services. 1992. *Healthy People 2000: National Health Promotion and Disease Prevention Objectives*. Boston: Jones and Bartlett.

U.S. Department of Health and Human Services, Administration for Children, Youth, and Families. 2009. *Child Maltreatment 2007*. Washington, DC: U.S. Government Printing Office.

Verbrugge, L. 1990. "Pathways of Health and Death," in *Women, Health and Medicine: A Historical Handbook*. R. Apple, ed. 41–79. New York: Garland.

Voeller, B. 1990. "Heterosexual Anal Intercourse: An AIDS Risk Factor," in *AIDS and Sex: An Integrated Biomedical and Biobehavioral Approach*. B. Voeller, J. Reinisch, and M. Gottlieb, eds. 276–311. New York: Oxford University Press.

Vogel, V. 1990. *American Indian Medicine*. Norman: University of Oklahoma Press.

Waber, R., B. Shiv, Z. Carmon, and D. Ariely. (2008). "Commercial Features of Placebo and Therapeutic Efficacy." *Journal of the American Medical Association* 299(9): 1016–17.

Wachter, R. 1999. "An Introduction to the Hospitalist Model." *Annals of Internal Medicine* 130: 4(Part 2): 338–42.

Waitzkin, H. 1985. "Information Giving in Medical Care." *Journal of Health and Social Behavior* 26(June): 81–101.

———. 2000. "Changing Patient-Physician Relationships in the Changing Health-Policy Environment," in *Handbook of Medical Sociology*, 5th ed. C. Bird and A. Fremont, eds. 271–83. Upper Saddle River, NJ: Prentice Hall.

———. 2001. *At the Front Lines of Medicine: How the Medical Care System Alienates Doctors and Mistreats Patients . . . and What We Can Do About it*. Lanham, MD: Rowman Littlefield.

Waldron, I. 1993. "Recent Trends in Sex Mortality Ratios for Adults in Developed Countries." *Social Science and Medicine* 36(4): 451–62.

———. 1994. "What Do We Know about Causes of Sex Differences in Mortality? A Review of the Literature," in *The Sociology of Health and Illness: Critical Perspectives*. P. Conrad and R. Kern, eds. 42–55. New York: St. Martin's Press.

Walker, A., and P. Parmar. 1993. *Warrior Marks: Female Genital Mutilation and the Sexual Blinding of Women*. New York: Harcourt Brace.

Walker, R. 1991. *AIDS Today, Tomorrow: An Introduction to the HIV Epidemic in America*. Atlantic Highlands, NJ: Humanities Press International.

Ward, D. 1993. "Women and the Work of Caring." *Second Opinion* 19(2): 11–25.

Ward, M. 1990. "The Politics of Adolescent Pregnancy: Turf and Teens in Louisiana," in *Births and Power: Social Change and the Politics of Reproduction*. W. Handwerker, ed. 147–64. San Francisco: Westview Press.

———. 1993a. "A Different Disease: AIDS and Health Care for Women in Poverty." *Culture, Medicine, and Psychiatry* 17(4): 413–30.

———. 1993b. "Poor and Positive: Two Contrasting Views from Inside the AIDS Epidemic." *Practicing Anthropology* 15(4): 59–61.

Wardwell, W. 1972. "Limited, Marginal, and Quasi-Practitioners," in *Handbook of Medical Sociology*. H. Freeman, S. Levine and L. Reeder, eds. 250–73. Englewood Cliffs, NJ: Prentice Hall.

Watkins, A. 1996. "Contemporary Context of Complementary and Alternative Medicine: Integrated Mind-Body Medicine," in *Fundamentals of Complementary and Alternative Medicine*. M. Micozzi, ed. 49–63. New York: Churchill Livingstone.

Watters, E. 2010. "The Americanization of Mental Illness." *New York Times Magazine*, January 8, 40–48.

Wedenoja, W., and E. Sobo. 1997. "Culture and Unconscious Motivation," in *Motivation and Culture*. D. Munro, J. F. Schumaker, and S. C. Carr, eds. 159–77. New York: Routledge.

Weinberg, M., and C. Williams. 1988. "Black Sexuality: A Test of Two Theories." *Journal of Sex Research* 25(2): 197–218.

Weinhold, B. 2006. "Epigenetics: The Science of Change." *Environmental Health Perspectives* 114(3): 160–67.

Weinstein, N. 1982. "Unrealistic Optimism about Susceptibility to Health Problems." *Journal of Behavioral Medicine* 5(4): 36–42.

———. 1989. "Perceptions of Personal Susceptibility to Harm," in *Primary Prevention of AIDS: Psychological Approaches*. V. Mays, G. Albee, and S. Schneider, eds. 142–67. Newbury Park, CA: Sage.

Weiss, G., and L. Lonnquist. 1994. *The Sociology of Health, Healing and Illness*. Englewood Cliffs, NJ: Prentice Hall.

———. 2003. *The Sociology of Health, Healing, and Disease*, 4th ed. Upper Saddle River, NJ: Prentice Hall.

Westat, Inc. 1988. *Study Findings: Study of National Incidence of Child Abuse and Neglect*. Washington, DC: U.S. Department of Health and Human Services.

Whiteford, M., and J. Friedl. 1992. *The Human Portrait: Introduction to Cultural Anthropology*, 3rd ed. Englewood Cliffs, NJ: Prentice Hall.

Whitehead, M. 1990. "The Health Divide," in *Inequalities in Health*. P. Townsend and N. Davidson, eds. 222–356. London: Penguin Books.

Widom, C. 1989. "The Cycle of Violence." *Science* 244(April): 160–66.

Wilensky, G., and D. Satcher. 2009. "Don't Forget about the Social Determinants of Health." *Health Affairs* 28(2): w194–98.

Williams, G., III. 1993. "Mind, Body, Spirit: The Dark Side of Hope: Seeing the Holes in the Holistic Movement." *Longevity* 28: 77–78.

Williams, R., Jr. 1970. *American Society: A Sociological Interpretation*. New York: Knopf.

Wilson, R. 1966. *Feminine Forever*. New York: M. Evans.

Wilson, W. 1987. *The Truly Disadvantaged*. Chicago: University of Chicago Press.

Wohl, S. 1984. *The Medical Industrial Complex*. New York: Harmony.

Wolf, N. 1991. *The Beauty Myth: How Images of Beauty Are Used Against Women*. New York: William Morrow.

Wootton, R., J. Craig, and V. Patterson, eds. 2006. *Introduction to Telemedicine*, 2nd ed. London: Royal Society of Medicine Press.

World Health Organization. 1994. *The Current Global Situation of the HIV/ AIDS Pandemic—Global Programme on AIDS Report*. Geneva: World Health Organization.

Worth, D. 1990. "Minority Women and AIDS: Culture, Race, and Gender," in *Cultural Aspects of AIDS*. D. Feldman, ed. 111–36. New York: Praeger.

Wyatt, S. B., D. R. Williams, R. Calvin, F. C. Henderson, E. R. Walker, and K. Winters. (2003). "Racism and Cardiovascular Disease in African Americans." *American Journal of the Medical Sciences* 325(6): 315–31.

Young, A. 1982. "The Anthropologies of Illness and Sickness." *Annual Reviews in Anthropology* 11: 257–85.

———. 1983. "The Relevance of Traditional Medical Cultures to Modern Primary Health Care." *Social Science and Medicine* 17(16): 1205–11.

———. 1986 [1976]. "Internalising and Externalising Medical Systems: An Ethiopian Example," in *Concepts of Health, Illness and Disease: A Comparative Perspective*. C. Currer and M. Stacey, eds. 139–60. Oxford: Berg.

Young, J., and L. Garro. 1994. *Medical Choice in a Mexican Village*, Reissue with changes. Prospect Heights, IL: Waveland.

Zborowski, M. 1952. "Cultural Components in Response to Pain." *Journal of Social Issues* 8: 16–30.

Zola, I. 1966. "Culture and Symptoms: An Analysis of Patients: Presenting Complaints." *American Sociological Review* 31: 615–30.

———. 1972. "Medicine as an Institution of Social Control." *Sociological Review* 20: 487–504.

———. 1983. *Socio-Medical Inquiries: Recollections, Reflections, and Reconsiderations*. Philadelphia: Temple University Press.

Index

About the Authors

Elisa J. Sobo, PhD, professor of anthropology at San Diego State University, began her career as a specialist in Caribbean health traditions. That work led to involvement in HIV/AIDS research, nutrition studies, and, most recently, health care quality improvement. Dr. Sobo's most recent book, *Culture and Meaning in Health Services Research: A Practical Field Guide*, combines ethnographic insight with methodological instruction and includes examples from real health services improvement projects. Internationally recognized for her contributions to the field, Dr. Sobo has served on the board of the Society for Medical Anthropology and on various journals' editorial boards. In addition to her work in academia, Dr. Sobo has worked directly in health care, including as an employee of Children's Hospital San Diego and with the Veterans Health Administration.

Martha O. Loustaunau, PhD, professor emerita of the Department of Sociology at New Mexico State University in Las Cruces, continues to teach online courses at New Mexico State in multicultural health care, medical ethics, and aging. Among her publications is the coedited volume *Life, Death, and In Between on the US-Mexico Border*. In addition to teaching and research and publication in academia, Dr. Loustaunau has worked directly in health care policy and administration; she served with the New Mexico Health Systems Agency for 10 years and was chair of the State Health Planning

Committee and Governing Body. She also served for several years with New Mexico Health Decisions, dealing with medical-ethical problems, and the Area Health Education Committee (AHEC), which supervises and awards grants for health education projects.